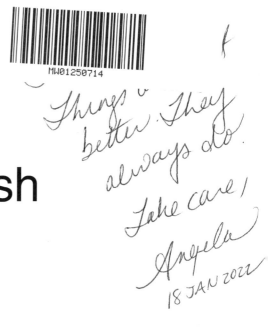

Flourish
or
Fade

A guide to total well-being
for women at midlife and beyond

Angela G. Gentile

Care to Age

Flourish or Fade:
A guide to total well-being
for women at midlife and beyond

Copyright © 2021 Angela G. Gentile

Special thanks to the *Sexuality Resource Education Centre Manitoba* for permission to use their definitions in the Sexual Wellness chapter.

DISCLAIMER: The information provided in this book is for educational purposes only and is not intended to replace the advice of your doctor, healthcare professional, financial advisor, or lawyer. You are encouraged to discuss any concerns you have with a qualified professional.

First Edition
ISBN-13: 979-8-7345-3179-2

Care to Age Press

Dedication

I dedicate this book to everyone I have worked with, talked with, interviewed, and gotten to know over the years. This includes my clients and their family members, my own family, including grandparents, parents, in-laws, and distant relatives (many have now passed on). It also includes the numerous mentors, teachers, co-workers, and employers I have enjoyed learning from. I would be remiss if I did not include the hundreds of women (and men) in my online communities. Without your openness and willingness to share, I could not have understood the complexities, challenges, and joys of growing older.

Acknowledgements

A wise person knows there is something
to be learned from everyone.

— Anonymous

Thank you to all who supported me over the years during my writing journey. This book has been years in the making, and I appreciate your patience and encouragement. This is the seventh attempt at writing a book on the subject. This time I finished it.

I am grateful for all of those who wrote on the subject before me. Your ideas and concepts have motivated me. Some of those books written by brilliant thought-leaders are mentioned in the back, under "Recommended Reading." Other books and references can be found sprinkled throughout the book.

Thank you to all my beta readers for their time, advice, suggestions, and encouragement: Virginia Wilson, Sheila Roy, Mary L. Beal, Agapito Gentile, Lorenzo Gentile, Dana MacLean, Marie Marley, Karen D. Austin, Andrea Moser, and Sherry Cels.

Special thanks to Nadine Jans for being my private cheerleader and coach. Your wise words and insightful advice have carried me through thick and thin. You are truly the best!

Thank you to the professionals involved such as Sue Lachman, of *Author Your Expertise*, and Frank Kresen of *Proof Positive*.

Thank you to my family and friends for being patient while I wrote, rewrote, took a break, and then promised to get back at it. Your unwavering support and faith in me are invaluable. Those who deserve special mention are Sheila Roy and Virginia Wilson.

Contents

You Weren't Born to Fade Away

Life may smooth away all of your rough edges, with its twists and turns and lessons to be learned.
Life may force you to fashion a tough outer shell.
Life may break you and reform you many many times until you don't even recognise the shapes you see in the mirror anymore.
And that's okay, it really is.
Just don't let life make you smaller.
Don't let anyone convince you that your cracks, your scars, are a sign of weakness.
They are war-wounds, my friend.
Battles fought and survived.
They are your story, your fight, your journey.
Let life reshape you over and over again, sure, but don't let it make you fade away.
Fading away is not what you are here for.
Let peace fill your heart as the years go by and your wisdom abounds.
Let anger and pettiness fall from its pedestal.
But don't let your voice diminish.
There are countless young women out there who need to hear you and hear you loudly.
You weren't put on this earth to burn brightly then fade away, my friend.
Get louder.
You have much more to say now.

— Donna Ashworth, author of *To The Women*

Preface

I have a passion for knowledge about living and aging well. Most books on aging are written by male doctors who take a very scientific approach with big words. I have read many of them. I have devoured all I can get my hands on but have not yet found the book written *for women by women*. So, I decided to write it. I started blogging in 2010 and have been working on this book since 2011!

I have worked with older adults (65+) since my kitchen-aide position in a personal care home when I was seventeen. I took on various jobs in the nursing home. I loved working with older adults so much that I decided on a career as a clinical social worker specializing in geriatrics.

I have heard and seen a lot over the years in many different roles as personal care home social worker, home care case coordinator, geriatric mental health clinician, and private-practice psychotherapist. I see how aging affects family members and friends. My collective knowledge and education on the subject of aging are extensive.

Early on, I realized not all older people go to nursing homes or need professional assistance. To me, old age was looking like a major case of doom and gloom. In order to balance out my skewed and unbalanced perspective of what growing old looked like, my interests naturally turned to studying healthy aging and "aging well." It was an innate need, a selfish one, in that I wanted to know what "successful" aging looked like. How could I live well and live long? Isn't that what everyone wants? I was curious about those who were SuperAgers. I wanted to learn the "secrets" to living long and well.

As the pendulum swung, I focused on the bright side of aging. Then I learned about ageism and its harmful effects. As I dug deeper, I realized that there could be *too much* positivity, creating harmful "positive ageism." This unwelcome pressure and high expectations of older people can cause poor self-esteem and other self-image problems. It can wear on a person's confidence. For example, we may expect older people to be wiser and more capable than they actually are. This can result in a person feeling "less than" or inadequate if they don't measure up to the elusive image of a "Successful Ager."

Having endured an anal-cancer diagnosis and treatment in 2017 at the age of 51 certainly changed my perspective. It is said one in two people will develop cancer in their lifetime. I consider getting old a privilege, as not everyone is fortunate enough to live long. I am cancer-free at the moment, but who knows what the future holds for me? There is a special place in my heart for all those who have endured a cancer ordeal or lost a loved one to this dreaded disease.

I have since adopted a "realistic yet optimistic" approach to growing old. It's what I advocate and strive for—a world free of elder abuse and the harmful effects of ageism and stereotyping. I envision a world where we can age and live well, on our own terms, free of external expectations and pressures. I hope and strive for a life that is most satisfying and enjoyable. I want that for you, too.

Now in my mid-50s, I have worked with hundreds, perhaps thousands, of older people. I have come to realize that healthy aging is more than just "functional ability." It is all-encompassing. This dynamic, fluid process is affected by genetics, environment, and our personal choices. This book presents my holistic approach to health based on the "wellness wheel" concept widely used in various health and educational settings. My method is called the *Flower of Wellness*, and it has been years in the making. I have applied this engaged, active aging philosophy to my life and will continue to do so until my dying day.

I have a special interest in women's issues. This book focuses on women's well-being at midlife and beyond; however, it will benefit anyone who reads it. It is based on a method that will help you find balance and overall wellness as you age. I believe striving for balance in all areas of your life can help you increase your happiness and life satisfaction. It may even help you live longer!

Aging is a lifelong process, but usually we don't see it that way. One day we wake up and feel like age has snuck up on us. Our aging experience doesn't seem like anyone else's. That's because it isn't. I have come to realize we get more heterogeneous the older we get. That is, we become more diverse, interesting, and unique as the years pass. Whether we are new-old (55+), young-old (65+), middle-old (75+), or old-old (85+), there is always something new to learn. We never stop learning!

Language matters. Ashton Applewhite, an anti-ageism advocate, suggests if we must use a term for older people, we should consider using "olders." I like that term, and I will also use "seniors" and "older adults" because those are the terms I feel are acceptable. In this book, anyone who is an "older" is someone 55 or better.

We "olders" have a lot of living to do. Let's make sure we are doing it in a way that makes us happy and healthy. As Applewhite observes, aren't you aging successfully if you woke up this morning?

This Book's Purpose

I present what I consider the 10 most essential dimensions (aspects) in life as we age and a guide to help you live a balanced life by examining your satisfaction in each of these dimensions. **Those 10 dimensions are Physical, Emotional, Brain, Social, Sexual, Spiritual, Environmental, Recreational, Financial, and Occupational.**

The information on each dimension is in no way exhaustive, as I know each topic I discuss could be a whole book in and of itself! I hope to get you thinking about the issues that affect your overall well-being and perhaps ignite a passion in you to learn more about the topics presented.

The goal is to help you make some positive changes in your life. What *you* think of as the most critical areas (dimensions) in your life may look different from what I am presenting here, and that's okay, too—the more personalized, the better. I will also provide you with two options on how to assess life satisfaction in all the areas and how you can improve them. One is a rating scale only, and the other is drawing a *Flower of Wellness*.

You may want to use the book as a selection for your book club (group discounts available; contact me). Perhaps it can be a catalyst for your life coaching, healing, self-development, or counselling journey. If you think of any new ideas for using this book, please email me at the address below.

I hope you enjoy reading this book. If you find it helpful, please consider telling your friends, putting it on social media, and posting a short review on Amazon and Goodreads. Word-of-mouth recommendations and online reviews are an author's best friend. They are much appreciated!

My wish for you is that, by my sharing this information, knowledge, past experiences, and wisdom with you, you can find a little something to take away to help you make the rest of your life the best of your life. I hope this book provides you with some new ideas and reinforces some good habits you have developed over the years. Active aging is a healthy and positive approach to living long and well. Instead of just fading away, let's flourish well into the winter of our lives.

Age well, my friend!

Angela G. Gentile
caretoage@gmail.com

How to Use This Book

Whatever's good for your soul, do that.

— Anonymous

Perhaps you picked up this book because you are looking for self-improvement or personal development. Maybe you are an "active ager" who strives for optimal health. You might be one of those people who wants to live to be 100—but doesn't want to get old. I assume you are like me—you would prefer to flourish in your later years rather than fade and disappear. No matter the reason, I'm glad you're here.

A healthy approach to maintaining vitality in the later years is a multidimensional concept. I have created a simple self-assessment tool for self-improvement—to help you feel better about yourself and get more satisfaction out of life. I call it the *Flower of Wellness* Method, which is based on 10 dimensions of well-being.

Increasing your life satisfaction can help you live longer. I will provide you with simple tips on how to motivate yourself and encourage others to live their best lives. You will be given suggestions on specific actions to improve your life and mindset regarding aging.

Change and improvement don't happen unless you are committed and decide to take charge of your life. Self-awareness is key. It starts with being curious, open, honouring your authentic self, and seeking joy. Sometimes it helps to have an accountability partner. We can do this together!

You may choose to read this book from start to finish, and that may be enough for you. Even if you get one tip that improves your life in some way, big or small, that is great. Or, you may choose to peruse the Contents and jump right to the topic area that you are most interested in.

If you choose to delve deeper, get yourself a journal, as each chapter comes with samples of *Questions* to ask yourself, *Affirmations* to consider, and *Things to Try*. Please note: Nothing will improve if you don't make any changes to your thoughts, feelings, attitudes, or behaviours. So, it does take *some* effort if you want to see progress!

Affirmations are statements that help change your thoughts and beliefs. (By the way, the queen of positive quotes and daily affirmations about self-love and acceptance was the late Louise Hay. You may have heard of her.) You can tweak the statements to suit yourself. To move towards your ideal life, I suggest saying them at least twice a day, morning and night, so that you start and end your day with positive thoughts.

There are many things you can try, and, hopefully, my suggestions will inspire some ideas of your own.

I will provide you with instructions on how to do the *Flower of Wellness* Method for Self-Assessment of Total Well-being in Chapter 13, entitled "How to Complete a Self-Assessment." There are two ways to assess where you are at—and one is for the more artistically inclined! The first is a score analysis (satisfaction rating from 1 to 4 for each dimension), and the second is the flower-diagram method. You may want to visit that chapter now and then come back here, to get an idea of how this process works.

Underlying Concepts Not Covered

Underlying and influencing each topic area (which will not be explored here in great depth) is our personality, values, morals, culture, and traditions. We are born with personality traits that help us express ourselves and drive the way we interact with others and our world. Our upbringing includes encouragement and discouragement, which shape our paths in this world. We are all unique when we consider our cultural and ethnic backgrounds.

Stories

Throughout the book, I have included stories from myself and others, as I believe we can learn a lot from real-life experiences. Instead of limiting myself to regurgitating information you can find elsewhere, these stories will help enhance your understanding and, in some cases, provide you with a little chuckle or added insight. Life is a series of events—including the good and the bad. We all have stories to share, and I have heard a lot!

Scientific Research

At other times, I will include scientific-research references at the end of each chapter. I believe in science, and, to help support some of the main points or statistics, I will include references as appropriate. If you come across something I have said that you believe is in error, offensive, ageist, or harmful, please let me know. I will fix it up for a future edition of this book.

I will include recommended readings, online resources, and a handy index to help enhance your reader experience.

No matter how you choose to use this book, I hope it provides you with some positive ideas to help you thrive in the second half of life.

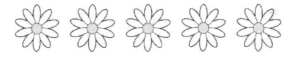

Reference

Zaninotto, P., Wardle, J., & Steptoe, A. (2016). Sustained enjoyment of life and mortality at older ages: analysis of the English Longitudinal Study of Ageing. *BMJ, 355*. doi: https://doi.org/10.1136/bmj.i6267. Cite as *BMJ* 2016; 355: i6267. Retrieved 14 Jan 2021.

Chapter 1

Embracing Aging

Do not resent growing old; many are denied the privilege.

— Irish Proverb

No one teaches us how to age. We learn from the media, our elders, and our personal experiences. Usually, our introduction to "old age" is when we are young and have grandparents in our lives. I was fortunate to have four grandparents up until I was twenty-nine. These natural intergenerational relationships were healthy and positive ones. I was able to witness firsthand the cycle of life. We are born, we grow up, we get old, and we die. I saw each of my grandparents go through the "old age and die" stage. They all lived into their eighties. I see growing old and dying as a natural part of life.

In addition to what we see in our own families and communities, we observe how older people are treated at work and, in turn, how olders act at work. Retirees may have different priorities from younger folks. Senior family members are perceived differently than the younger ones. Our older relatives have a wealth of history, stories, and "ways of life" that are different from our own. Our intergenerational relationships in our workplaces, communities, and families can help us become more understanding of the other generations' needs.

When Does Midlife Start?

Some people ask me, "When does midlife start?" That's a good question. I think the answer is within ourselves. It's subjective. If we don't feel "young" anymore, yet we don't feel "old," I would think that would mean we are in our "middle" years. For some women it may start at menopause. Midlife may last well into our sixties! I know for myself, at 55, I identified with the "new-old," because I qualified for senior discounts. I don't "feel" old, but I am certainly not young. Midlife started for me around 40.

Aging Well—Total Well-Being

Aging well (and living well) encompasses more than just the physical aspects. It's more than "active aging." Women, especially, get caught up in the physical-looks department (beauty, wrinkle-free skin, and body weight). In North American society, it is very easy to slip into that trap. Sure, body image is a big part of our lives. I don't deny that. What I want to emphasize here is that there is more to it.

Ageism

In North American society, we are bombarded with ageist or anti-aging messages that are ultimately harmful. Our culture is obsessed with youth and beauty. Older people are sometimes valued less in our society (the COVID-19 pandemic exposed this tragedy), and it should not be this way. I strongly advocate for valuing each individual—no matter what age they are. If we don't, we are only hurting our future selves (if we are gifted with living a long life). If we change our attitudes and enhance the way we age, we can embrace the process. If enough of us (and I know there are a few!) speak up, speak out, and encourage others, we can shift a whole generation of people who will celebrate and revere old age. We are learning how not to be ageist; now, we have to learn how to be anti-ageist.

Age Accelerators

There is only one proven way to *stop* growing older, and most of us say we don't prefer that alternative. Growing older is a natural process. There will be normal genetic wear and tear on aging skin, hair, joints, bones, organs, etc. The aging process is normal, and these are non-modifiable changes and deterioration. For example, how do you *stop* your hair from greying? Learning how to accept these changes is a big task for some of us. (You *can* dye your hair, though!)

Extrinsic factors and lifestyle factors can make you feel like you are aging more quickly than you would have if these things were not in your life. Age-accelerators can hasten the aging process and may even shorten our lifespan. There are modifiable factors (things within our control). We need to learn what those things are. It will be different for everyone.

For example, thinning hair is a genetic condition. There will be people who can't do anything about it. On the other hand, hair can fall out because the person is under tremendous emotional stress. If we remove the stress, the hair will become full and healthy again. My hair thinned when I was undergoing immense stress. I was also undergoing chemotherapy and radiation at the time, so once I got through that, my hair eventually grew back.

Aging is inevitable. Take charge of the way you age to lessen its impact.

We live our lives as if we will live forever. Some of us take a more proactive approach to illness prevention, and we take heed. There are lifestyles we choose that are healthy and those that are less healthy.

Take smoking, for example. Some people smoke, and although there are warnings everywhere (including the packaging), people continue to smoke. I have heard my brother call cigarettes "cancer sticks," as we all know they increase the risk of developing cancer. Even secondhand smoke is dangerous. One 91-year-old woman I talked to said, "It doesn't really matter if you smoke or not. Some people live well into their later years even though they smoke. It doesn't mean you are guaranteed a cancer diagnosis. It just increases your risk." When we encounter conflicting advice like this, it makes it hard to follow the experts' advice.

We also know that a sedentary lifestyle—think "couch potato"—also puts you at a higher risk for developing health problems. In 2002, the World Health Organization warned that physical inactivity is a leading cause of disease and disability. Decades later, this is still the case, and, sadly, people are not taking heed. The U.S. Department of Health and Human Services (HHS.gov) reports only 33% of adults meet the physical-activity recommendations. Shockingly, only 33% of children are physically active every day. I believe and understand that even if you stand up once every 30 to 60 minutes or so, it is better for your health than sitting and doing nothing (excuse me while I stand up and stretch for a bit—you should, too!).

Following is a list of age accelerators, which are modifiable by lifestyle choices.

Age Accelerators:

- Too much unprotected exposure to the sun
- Smoking
- Sedentary lifestyle (too much sitting or long periods of inactivity)
- Problematic use of alcohol or drugs
- Overeating/unhealthy diet/lack of staying properly hydrated
- Loneliness
- Inadequate amount of sleep
- Stress
- Holding anger and resentment
- Negative attitude towards aging
- Refusal to accept the changes that come with aging
- Refusing to wear hearing aids or glasses
- Wrong assumptions of what is "inevitable"
- Loss of purpose
- Limitations we put on ourselves due to "our age"
- Harmful ageist stereotyping

Knowing what those age-accelerators are and applying a systems approach to total well-being can help you live a long, happy, and contented life. I will show you how you can do this by using the *Flower of Wellness* Method designed for women at midlife and beyond.

The *Flower of Wellness*

I first learned of the "wellness wheel" method years ago, when I went to see a counsellor during a stressful time in my life. To feel whole, balanced, and content, I learned that I needed to take a closer look at all areas of my life—body, mind, and soul. She had me complete an exercise that included a closer look at several areas of my life, such as physical, career, spiritual, emotional, etc. I remember taking the time to fill out that questionnaire, and I realized at the time I didn't have any recreational or leisure activities. I didn't understand what spirituality really was. The counsellor shed light on what I didn't even know I was missing. She pointed out where my life was out of balance and what I needed to do to feel more balanced. The tool she used with me was designed for younger adults. This experience planted a seed in me, which I have nourished over the years.

Years later, after revisiting this "balanced" approach to well-being, I couldn't find anything geared to those in middle-to-later years. I also noticed that sexuality wasn't addressed in the way it should be. I have since developed a wellness-wheel approach that is very comprehensive and includes the issues that come with aging. I call it the *Flower of Wellness*, and, for this book, I have tailored it to women at midlife and beyond.

Bloomers take charge of the way they age by pursuing fulfillment and satisfaction throughout their lives.

I encourage you to embrace aging with all its wonder, challenges, and opportunities.

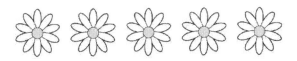

References

Myers, J. E., Sweeney, T. J., & Witmer, J. M. (2000). The wheel of wellness counseling for wellness: A holistic model for treatment planning. *Journal of Counseling & Development*, 78(3), 251.

Myers, J. E., & Sweeney, T. J. (2005). The indivisible self: An evidence-based model of wellness (reprint). *Journal of Individual Psychology*, 61(3), 269-279.

Chapter 2

Flower of Wellness
for Total Well-Being

If I had my life to live over again, I'd pick more daisies.

— Nadine Stair

I first learned of a holistic approach to health and wellness in my social-work training. This is also known as a total-wellness approach—body, mind, and soul. In social work, we consider the whole person, considering all the influences in their life—"Systems Theory." We do what is called a "holistic assessment." For example, if a mother comes to us saying her son is unmanageable, we take a look at all the factors that affect the child. We look at his social life, school life, home life, physical health, mental health, diet, stress factors, etc. What appears initially to be a problem with the "person" often turns out to be the result of many different factors. Maybe the boy is stressed because he is being bullied at school, and perhaps he gets irritated and yells a lot because he has stomach pains due to lactose intolerance. Also, his parents have been talking to him about their decision to get a divorce. Think of a holistic approach as looking at the whole person, including *all* the influencing factors. For this boy, his stomach ailments (physical), home life (social), and school life (occupation) are all impacting his feelings and, ultimately, his behaviour. All of these factors work together as a system. As a helper, we can identify inefficiencies or missing pieces—resulting in corrections or enhancements—which can help the person become whole and balanced.

Family therapy, individual counselling, changes to the environment, and other strategies can help the system recover. Once the system is repaired, the person is happier, and things run more smoothly (until the next difficulty comes along, and it will!). The systems approach is helpful at any age, throughout our lifespan, especially as we grow older.

Why the Need for a Holistic Approach to Aging?

A total-wellness approach to life will help you determine what areas (if any) need more attention to help you live a balanced, satisfactory, and happy life. You will learn where there is room to grow. If you are new to this concept of total well-being, you may discover missing elements—essential parts of your life that you didn't even know you had hiding in the shadows. A holistic approach will confirm you are on the right track to living a long and fulfilling life. It will also help you develop the resilience needed to carry you through any tough times.

Flower of Wellness Method

After years of researching, learning, growing, and maturing, I found myself going back to that time with the counsellor, years ago. I thought about Systems Theory and put together an overall wellness plan. I tested it out with myself and others. This led to creating a total-wellness self-assessment tool that has shown to be helpful to those who are middle-aged and beyond. I love taking photos of flowers and growing flowers in my garden, so it was only natural for me to choose a flower (think "daisy") rather than a wheel or a pie. The *Flower of Wellness* Method I am introducing in this book is a modified version of the wellness wheel, specifically designed for today's woman at midlife and beyond.

The *Flower of Wellness* and Ten Dimensions

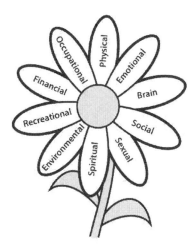

The *Flower of Wellness* has 10 petals, each representing one of the 10 dimensions of wellness, which I have found to be of utmost significance in our lives if we want balance, especially as we age:

Ten Dimensions of Wellness:

1. Physical
2. Emotional
3. Brain
4. Social
5. Sexual
6. Spiritual
7. Environmental
8. Recreational
9. Financial
10. Occupational

All of the dimensions are interconnected. There are multiple layers, and the connections are often intricate and complicated. They are not mutually exclusive of each other. These areas of your life are dynamic—not static—becoming more important to you during certain times in your life. Other areas may remain dormant and a non-issue.

Each dimension is presented in a silo of sorts, but in real life, each area will influence and touch on the other. Sometimes many issues will overlap and connect at the same time. It can be complicated. These overlapping and interconnected facets of our mind, body, and soul (and more!) are interdependent. For example, a cancer diagnosis can affect our Emotional and Sexual well-being (I know, as I was diagnosed with anal cancer and treated with chemoradiation in 2017). Memory impairment can affect our Social life and our Occupation. Retirement can affect our Financial status and Emotional health. So, it is crucial to consider how each element influences the other. Underlying our ability to cope with life's changes and challenges is our innate resilience and level of self-compassion.

Resilience

Resilience is the ability to "bounce back" after getting knocked down. Sometimes we can get back up quicker than other times, depending on what else is going on in our lives. Having a strong, healthy body, a healthy emotional and mental outlook, and a spiritual connection can help you be resilient. Sometimes life will look different after a major crisis (such as the loss of a loved one or getting a cancer diagnosis), but getting back to a new kind of normal is part of life. I know this from personal experience. Life is full of challenges, losses, setbacks, and strains. I believe these experiences help us become more compassionate and understanding towards others experiencing similar situations. I also think it helps us learn to be more accepting of others and appreciate things that are going well in our own lives.

Self-compassion

Another healthy mindset has to do with self-compassion. Most of us never learned about this concept. We have been taught not to think of ourselves—instead put others first. Self-compassion is a concept we can work on as we age. Self-compassion is the ability to be kind, accepting, and patient with ourselves. Most of us know how to be kind to a friend. We know what needs to be said or done to make that person feel better. Sadly, we haven't been taught how to be compassionate towards ourselves. We can be very critical. Our negative self-talk can be continuous, ultimately harming our self-esteem. Low self-esteem can lead to negative coping strategies, such as problem drinking or overeating, or the opposite, starving ourselves. I would encourage you to be more self-compassionate and to be patient with the process. There is no prize for racing to the finish line, and things usually don't change overnight.

One little way to be more compassionate towards yourself is to pay attention to your thoughts. For example, if you are cooking and you end up spilling more salt into the pot than you wanted, you may end up saying to yourself, "I'm so stupid. I saw that coming. The top has fallen off before. Why didn't I remember that?" Now imagine it was a good friend who did the same thing. You witnessed her adding salt to the pot, and the top and a bunch more salt fell into the pot. What would you say to her? Would you say, "You are so stupid. You should have seen that coming..."? No, you would probably say, "Oh, well—accidents happen. That's okay. Let's try and fix that." We tend to be more compassionate towards people we care about. Self-compassion is learning how to care about ourselves more—in turn helping us feel happier and more at ease. We tend to be harder on ourselves because we don't want to become complacent and lazy. What ends up happening is we harm our sense of self and risk becoming sad and depressed.

Why a Holistic Approach is Beneficial

A holistic approach to aging will help make you feel more balanced, settled, and at peace. This program will give you some control over how you age. Instead of sitting back, being passive, and growing old (that is, taking a seat in "God's Waiting Room"), you can make some active and sound decisions on how to live your life. As a counsellor, coach, and mentor, I will teach you how to deal with whatever curveball may be thrown at you.

Sure, sometimes life will get you down. Life is full of those moments. These experiences are necessary so that we can be more grateful for those times when things are going well. Since I have been practicing a balanced approach to life and aging, I have been more resilient and capable. As a middle-aged woman, I feel stronger and wiser every day.

Take a Closer Look, and Embrace Aging

Instead of ignoring the signs and symptoms of aging (thereby denying and dishonouring ourselves and our future selves), I encourage you to take a closer look at where you are. To enjoy a balanced life, consider each dimension and maximize it to your satisfaction. I believe we all have the power to make those changes and to ride the waves as they come. Adapting, accommodating, and being resilient to life's challenges will help us get through this adventure we call life. Plus, a good attitude towards aging goes a long way!

Some people have told me that they would never do a self-assessment, and that's okay with me, too. Some people choose to take one day at a time. This program is designed for those who want to embrace aging and make the most out of life—body, mind, and soul. Let's start with learning a little more about each dimension. Then I will provide you with the instructions on how to complete a self-assessment.

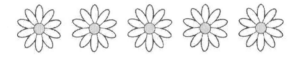

References

Diaz, K. M., Howard, V. J., Hutto, B., Colabianchi, N., Vena, J. E., Safford, M. M., Blair S. N., & Hooker, S. P. (2017). Patterns of Sedentary Behavior and Mortality in U.S. Middle-Aged Older Adults: A National Cohort Study. *Annals of Internal Medicine*, 167(7). https://doi.org/10.7326/M17-0212. Retrieved 14 Jan 2021.

U.S. Department of Health and Human Services. Healthy People. Available at: https://www.cdc.gov/nchs/healthy_people/index.htm. Retrieved 15 Feb 2021.

Chapter 3

Physical Wellness

It is health that is the real wealth,
and not pieces of gold and silver.

— Mahatma Gandhi

Health is wealth. When I think of this statement, I automatically think of physical well-being. I believe that the concept of health involves so much more than that. Our mental health is just as important as our physical health, yet some tend to stigmatize and avoid the issues surrounding mental illness and disability. I will leave the topics surrounding mental health for the chapters on emotional and brain wellness. Physical well-being is a huge topic, and what I want to share here is what I feel is most pertinent for women at midlife and beyond.

NOTE: I am not a licensed physician, however, I have worked in the healthcare field as a clinical social worker for more than 25 years. This includes 11 years working as a geriatric clinician, consulting with geriatric psychiatrists (doctors who specialize in working with older adults who have mental-health problems). My suggestions and thoughts here are mainly for your own education and awareness. Please discuss any concerns you may have with your licensed healthcare provider before making any changes that will affect your health and well-being. I also encourage you to consult medical professionals and specialists to help you with preventative and curative care for chronic and terminal diseases.

Longevity (Living Long)

I read about the Blue Zones a few years ago, and I was intrigued. These are areas in the world where people live the longest. One of those areas is in Nicoya, Costa Rica. I traveled there in 2015 and saw older people walking along the roads and working in their gardens. I was told the people in Nicoya keep active and eat a diet rich in fresh fruits and vegetables. On the way through one of the towns, I saw a very tanned and lean older man walking along the road. I asked our tour guide, "How old do you think that man is?" He responded, "He's probably older than one hundred. He was an old man when I was young." This experience drove home the notion that keeping active and eating lots of fruits and vegetables is key to longevity and helped confirm for me what we are learning from the Blue Zones.

Ideal Body Weight

What is the ideal body weight? During our lifespan, most of us will see some ups and downs in our weight. Stress, poor dietary habits, lack of physical activity, hormonal changes, and other factors can impact our weight—ultimately impacting our health. For a guide on healthy body weight, the Body Mass Index (BMI) Calculator is often used. Search for "BMI calculator" on the internet. You will find an easy way to determine if you are underweight, normal weight, overweight, or obese. You just have to know your height and weight. Some of the fancier calculators also include gender and age. Some people don't like using BMI as a gauge, but I have found it very helpful as a general guide.

Some experts report that it's better to have a little extra weight on us for protection factors as we get older. The BMI targeted range tends to shift toward the right, especially after age 80. The extra pounds can help provide protection in case we become ill, have dental issues, or have a fall. I know the importance of this, as I lost 30 pounds during a health crisis. When I went through cancer treatment, I was grateful for my extra weight at the time. Having a low BMI puts you at risk for frailty, so it's important to keep up our weight, even if it means using nutritional supplements. The maintenance of muscle mass and strong bones through exercise and walking also offers added protection against frailty.

For extra motivation, you can purchase a "smart" digital bathroom scale. I have one that has a companion app, and it keeps track of many different aspects of my body composition. These scales are variable in quality and accuracy, and, in addition to tracking weight and BMI, they claim to measure additional components such as body fat, body water, bone mass, visceral fat, body age, protein, basal metabolism, skeletal muscle, and subcutaneous fat. Readings are displayed in different colours, with red indicating areas for improvement or "risk," such as a higher-than-average body-fat composition. It's a visual to tell you what you need to work on. The app records all the data so you can see trends.

It can also be helpful to record your weight in a diary or electronic notes record. An accountability partner helps motivate and encourage. Walking buddies make exercising more fun. Setting goals with someone and sharing your progress can help you meet your targets.

Waist circumference is also an important indicator to determine if you have an unhealthy amount of visceral fat that surrounds your organs inside your abdomen (intra-abdominal fat). The term "Beer Belly" is often used to describe a person who has an average build but a large, round stomach. It is usually a sign of having an unhealthy diet and not enough physical activity. The Mayo Clinic states if you have more weight above your hips, you are at greater risk of heart disease and type 2 diabetes. Use a fabric or body tape measure to determine the circumference just above your hips. To help reduce risks to your health, the World Health Organization recommends women should strive for a waist circumference of 31 inches (78.7 cm) or less, and men, 34.5 inches (87.6 cm) or less. Note: Dual-energy X-ray absorptiometry (DEXA scan) can measure bone density, muscle mass, and intra-abdominal fat.

Sleep and Sleep Hygiene

How do we start our day? Ideally, we would wake up after a long, deep, refreshing sleep. How disappointing it is to have to start our day after a night of fitful slumber. Sleep is necessary to give us the energy and clarity needed to take on a new day. As adults, we need between six and eight hours of sleep daily. If we have trouble sleeping, we need to look at our habits and make adjustments until we reach a solution. Sometimes it means we need to cut back on the caffeine or spend more time awake during the daylight hours. For those who can't sleep due to hormonal reasons (hot flashes), we may need to turn on a fan or change our sleepwear to something lighter and 100% cotton. Some sleep with one leg out! Or, open a window when it's cool outside. A new pillow, mattress, sheets, or blankets may help. Sometimes medication can be prescribed to help calm our "monkey mind."

I'm a morning person and a night person.
So, I have to be a nap person,
or else I'm a tired person.

— Jeri Smith-Ready, *Wicked Game*

A bedtime routine is just as important now as it was when we were younger. Find what works for you. Perhaps you need to cut back on screen time (computer, tablet, phone, television) at night—and instead, read (not too stimulating, though!), listen to music, or do crossword puzzles. If you have a cuddle buddy (the furry or human type!), get some snuggles in. Take a warm bath or shower—anything to calm your thinking. Coming out of a warm shower causes a decrease in body temperature, which can be calming. If all else fails, you may need to try Cognitive Behavioural Therapy for insomnia (CBTi). Sleep disorders can also cause problems, so it's important to talk to a doctor if you don't feel like you are getting enough rest.

A few years back, I was going through a lot of stress at work which caused me to have difficulty sleeping. The environment was very stressful, and I lacked sleep due to the worry and pressures. I remember becoming very disoriented due to the lack of sleep. Fortunately, the situation was resolved, and I was able to get back to a regular sleep pattern.

If you have serious sleep issues, you may want to seek out a sleep specialist. It's important to seek advice from a licensed medical professional to identify treatable or reversible conditions that may be contributing to sleep disruption such as sleep apnea, pain, heart problems, mental-health issues, and others. A licensed physician who is a sleep specialist has received additional training in sleep medicine. A licensed sleep specialist psychologist focuses on the mental-health and behavioural aspects related to problems with sleep. If you have sleep apnea or other sleep-related issues caused by breathing or other structural problems, you may want to seek out help from an otolaryngologist (ear, nose, and throat specialist). Always seek advice from a licensed medical professional when it comes to problems with sleep.

Diet and Personalized Nutrition

We can't survive without air, food, and water. Breathing happens naturally, whether it's a quick, shallow breath or a long, deep one. Take a moment now, and take a big deep breath, just like I did as I wrote this! We can't live without air. Nutrition and hydration form the basis of the fuel we need to keep our bodies functioning. We can live longer without food than we can without water. I find my body needs at least 6-8 glasses of water or liquids (such as juice or green tea) daily to feel adequately hydrated.

Over the years, I have interviewed many "tea and toast" ladies. These are the women who have tea and toast for breakfast—and have done so for years. I know my grandmother and other relatives did. It's an easy breakfast but not the greatest for nutritional content. If it's not toast and jam, popular alternatives maybe a crumpet, muffin, Danish, tart, or Chelsea bun. I remember going to hotels that serve a "Continental Breakfast." It's usually a light breakfast meal consisting of these pastries and other baked goods. I would suggest looking at the nutritional content of the first meal of the day and making sure it's not all food with high sugar content.

There are many different approaches to healthy nutrition. However, I keep coming back to the meal plans that stress the importance of plant-based foods (e.g., fruits, vegetables, grains, nuts, legumes), especially dark and colourful fruits and veggies such as spinach, peppers, zucchini, and blueberries.

The *Canada Food Guide* (food-guide.canada.ca/en/) places an emphasis on "plenty of vegetables and fruits, protein, whole grains, and water." (The *Guide* is available in many languages.)

17

In addition to the *Canada Food Guide*, the general nutrition plans that I endorse for optimal well-being include the Mediterranean Diet, Dietary Approaches to Stop Hypertension (DASH), and the MIND diet. The Mediterranean Diet is styled after the cuisine found along the Mediterranean Sea, such as that in Spain, Italy, and France. It is a diet rich in vegetables, fruits, whole grains, beans, nuts, seeds, and olive oil. The DASH diet's heart-healthy focus is designed to help reduce or control high blood pressure. Similar to the Mediterranean Diet, DASH is also rich in vegetables and fruits.

However, it has an additional emphasis on foods that have higher calcium, potassium, and magnesium content, at the same time avoiding choices that are higher in sodium. MIND combines the two and focuses on brain health, which, in effect, wards off dementia and poor cognitive function.

> Cut back on sugary sweets and drinks. Sugar is addictive and has detrimental effects. It has no nutritional value. It is linked to tooth decay, inflammation, heart disease, and many other medical problems.

Tips for Healthy Eating:

- Be sure to eat foods rich in antioxidants, such as fruits, vegetables, whole grains, and nuts.
- The more colourful the vegetable, the better (e.g., red bell peppers, sweet potatoes).
- When choosing green, leafy vegetables, the darker the better (e.g., spinach, kale).
- Limit your consumption of red meat.
- The more active you are the more protein you need to build and repair muscle.
- Choose healthy fat sources such as fish, avocado, and olive oil.
- Cut back on sweets and junk food.
- Eat a variety of healthy foods every day.
- Choose organic when possible.

- Make water your beverage of choice.
- Cook at home more often.
- Read nutrition labels.
- Slow down and enjoy your food.
- Eat with others whenever possible.

If you are interested in the latest news on health and nutrition, check out Dr. Michael Greger's work. Diets that are heavy on plant-based choices, clean eating—whole and natural foods—and light on the processed foods are sure to be winners!

A balanced approach to eating well with attention to drinking plenty of water is key to a healthy body weight. Being mindful of how much you are eating results in attention to caloric intake. Many of us are too familiar with overindulging. To put it plain and simple: Most of us eat too much! If you aren't sure of your "Basal Metabolic Rate," you can find a BMR calculator online. This will tell you how many calories your body needs at rest. Please remember, if you are going to try any new diet or approach, please review with your healthcare provider first. A dietician can help you identify your individualized nutritional needs.

Food diaries can be very useful, as they help us become aware of what we are eating. Mindful eating is another approach. Many of us eat without really thinking about it. Mindful eating requires us to be more conscious of our actions, the taste of the food, the signal that we are full. The concept of being more "mindful of our eating habits" is so important that The *Canada Food Guide* has recommended it.

Everything in moderation (and not too much!) tends to work in the long run. A healthy, balanced diet suited to your medical dietary needs is what all registered dieticians (RD) recommend. Consult with a registered dietician or nutritionist if you have specific concerns about your health and dietary needs.

Personalized nutrition is a new way of approaching how we eat. It sometimes takes a lot of trial and error. As we age, things can change. Become aware of how your body and gut feel after you have eaten certain foods. For example, some people say they have problems with nightshades. Others can't tolerate greasy food, and we are learning more about gluten sensitivity. There are emerging genetic tests (very personalized) that claim to identify your individual food intolerances based on DNA analysis. It is anticipated that we will learn more about the applicability and accuracy of these tests over the coming years.

As we age, our body metabolizes foods and medicines differently. We can even develop allergies and sensitivities that we never had before. I have noticed I am more sensitive to caffeine. I am okay when I have a drink of regular tea, but if I have a second cup, I feel my heart racing. I have cut down on drinking tea, so now I try to have decaffeinated or herbal instead. Also important to keep in mind is that caffeine in tea and coffee is a stimulant, which can actually worsen anxiety. So, it's best to cut back where possible.

There are lots of different cooking appliances and tools we can use to make nutritious, home-cooked meals. In addition to the conventional cooking appliances such as a stove, oven, and microwave, don't forget about these other devices that you may or may not use on a daily basis:

Cooking Appliances:

- Slow cooker
- Pressure cooker
- Wok
- Dehydrator
- Air Fryer
- Steamer
- Convection oven
- Barbecue

There are tons of recipes on the internet and guidelines on how to cook with the tools mentioned above. Get creative, and have fun!

Food is a major part of our lives. Depending on your body and your needs, you may have some digestive issues that tend to get more pronounced as you age. I will share some of my stories here in case it helps you or someone you know.

Elimination (Pooping and Peeing)

Many older people I know are fixated on their bowel habits. It's a horrible feeling to be constipated, but there are ways around this that can help. Some medications can cause our bowels to move slowly (e.g., painkillers such as morphine or codeine), which is hard to prevent if you rely on these drugs to control your pain. It is important to inform your primary care provider if you are experiencing changes in your bowel patterns, constipation, or loose stools, as there may be an underlying condition contributing to this that requires additional investigation. If you are prone to getting constipated, you may be able to manage your problem with diet and exercise. Prunes, prune juice, oatmeal, fibre, nuts, and other foods can help people stay regular. Making sure you are drinking enough water and getting some exercise can also help. There are medications that can prevent and treat constipation, and you should review with your healthcare provider what is recommended for you.

Some older women tend to get more urinary tract infections (UTI) or bladder infections than others. Symptoms can include frequency and a burning sensation when urinating. If you feel you may have a UTI, it's essential to get it checked by a healthcare professional. It's an easy test. A sample of urine is sent to the lab and examined. Antibiotics can be prescribed, and the UTI usually goes away in a few days. (Make sure you check with the doctor or pharmacist about mixing alcohol with antibiotics, as sometimes that can interfere with the antibiotic's effectiveness.)

Urinary dribbling or incontinence is also common in women. Women can wear a panty-liner in their underwear for stress incontinence (leaking when you laugh, cough, or have to go urgently!), or they can wear a full-on incontinent brief if needed. The pull-up styles are like panties, so they aren't embarrassing at all. People won't even know you have them on. However, if there is a sudden onset of urinary incontinence or worsening symptoms, talk to a healthcare professional. You may also benefit from a pelvic-floor physiotherapist and be given some treatment or pelvic-floor exercises to strengthen your muscles "down below," including Kegels.

Irritable Bowel Syndrome

I have been living with irritable bowel syndrome (IBS) since I was in my early twenties. In my fifties, after a bout of anal cancer and treatment with chemoradiation, I was no longer willing or able to deal with my IBS. My gut health was suffering, and I wanted to get down "to the bottom of it." After seeing a gastroenterologist for my bowel issues (cramping, bloating, pain, diarrhea), he suggested I try a "Low-FODMAP elimination diet" while waiting weeks for an appointment for a scope up the butt. I did some Googling and then downloaded the "Monash University FODMAP Diet" app (created in Australia). I learned there are two types of IBS. One is IBS-D, where the "D" stands for "diarrhea." The other is IBS-C, where the "C" is short-form for "constipation."

I got serious about tackling my IBS-D problem, and it took me only a few weeks to learn I am sensitive to foods with galactooligosaccharides (GOS). This includes wheat, cashews, pistachios, and chickpeas. I have completely changed my diet, and my IBS is now under control. If you have any gut or bowel problems, personalized nutrition can help change your life for the better.

Pelvic Organ Prolapse

Pelvic organ prolapse is a best-kept secret. That's where the uterus, bladder, small intestine, or rectum protrudes into the vaginal wall which can cause other problems. Common symptoms experienced include pressure (or bulging) in the vaginal canal, urinary incontinence, fecal incontinence, and painful intercourse. One in two women over the age of 50 will be affected by pelvic organ prolapse. Something not right "down there"? Don't suffer in silence. Talk about it with your friends. End the stigma. See your doctor and discuss options that are right for you.

Vitamins and Supplements

Most, if not all, of our nutritional needs can be met through a healthy, balanced diet. As we age, however, our bodies change, and the way we process our food can change. There are some supplements that may be recommended, or your healthcare provider may recommend a blood test to identify if you have any vitamin deficiencies. Your doctor may recommend a vitamin as a treatment to prevent progression of chronic disease such as lutein for age-related macular degeneration. Other vitamins include but are not limited to vitamin D and vitamin B12. When searching online, I usually check out the Mayo Clinic website. They have tons of information on all kinds of health topics (such as Vitamin B12), and they keep it updated with the latest research. The Mayo Clinic Staff reviews it, and it includes trustworthy scientific references.

Not all vitamins and supplements are alike and vary in quality, dosage, route (e.g., swallow, chewable, melt under the tongue), and pricing. Some supplements and medications should not be taken together, so it's best to talk to a healthcare professional to find out what would be best for you.

Concerning Vitamin D, we know that we get a good dose of it from sunshine. Our skin makes Vitamin D when it is exposed to sunlight. But we also know we can get skin cancer from *too much* sun. The literature I have read states that we still get the benefits of Vitamin D even when we wear sunscreen—and 15 minutes of sunshine daily is all we need to help keep us healthy.

Medications

Many of us are prescribed pharmaceuticals (medication) for different ailments. People with diabetes may have to take medicine to help maintain healthy insulin levels. People who are at risk for a stroke may have to take heart medicine. Achy joints caused by arthritis may get so bad that your doctor or nurse

Take outdated medications back to the pharmacy for destruction and safe disposal.

practitioner may prescribe an anti-inflammatory. I believe in an integrative approach to health and wellness. This means using the best that science offers in terms of conventional medicine, combined with safe and natural alternatives and complementary treatments. For example, when my arthritis flares up, I may have to take a pain reliever (analgesic) or topical rub to take the edge off, but I will also try some gentle stretches and a heating pad. This combination usually helps me get some relief from the pain I feel in my lower back.

A word about safe medication use: Keep an accurate and updated list of your prescriptions and the condition they are prescribed for, including all over-the-counter (OTC) medications you take on a regular basis. Sometimes there are potential interactions between OTC and prescription medications. Bring this list with you to appointments with your healthcare provider.

Consider discussing with your pharmacy dispensing methods such as pill packs (bubble packs), a dosette (pill organizer), or easy-to-open bottles if you are finding it difficult to keep track of the medications prescribed. I have seen people who have made a little chart; they check it off when they have taken their medication. Do what works.

Doctor Visits

Your health needs and general well-being will help dictate how often you should see a healthcare practitioner. Some people like to see the doctor annually for a physical (e.g., blood-sugar tests, a blood-pressure measurement, breast exam, or pap test) to help screen for any potential health problems. Certain tests will or won't be included, depending on your age.

I received notices in my mailbox in my fiftieth year suggesting I should have a mammogram (breast x-ray) and a colon check. My doctor and pharmacist both advised me of the shingles vaccine and told me I should consider this as well. My doctor also recommends the annual flu shot, and, in addition, I received the new-to-the-scene COVID-19 vaccine. It is anticipated that the COVID-19 vaccine will also become part of a recommended immunization series although the frequency is not yet known. Depending on where you live, you may or may not receive these kinds of notices. My friend Sherry, at age 70, was told by her doctor that pap tests are no longer included in her annual checkup.

In Canada, we have a government-funded healthcare system that pays for most of the costs of primary and specialist care, access to allied healthcare professionals (e.g., social work, physiotherapy), investigations, tests, and hospitalizations. Coverage of medications varies across the country, with many provinces providing medication coverage to older adults and high-risk populations. The government programs are very keen on catching age-related issues early on to reduce healthcare costs down the line (at the same time helping keep us healthy).

If you take medication, you will want to make sure you know what you are taking, what you are taking it for, what side effects to watch for, and how long to take the medication. Not all medication is good for us, and some come with risks. This is especially important as we age. A list called the "Beers Criteria" (not the drink) was put out by the American Geriatrics Society. This is a list of potentially inappropriate medications older adults (65+) should avoid. It is updated every few years. It is surprising to learn how many drugs are deemed potentially inappropriate.

If you are taking medications, your doctor will advise you how long you should take the medication for. You may also want to have a medication review with a pharmacist. There may be some medications you no longer require, and you can discuss this with your physician. If you still need to take a lot of drugs (called "polypharmacy") and want help keeping them organized, you can get a little dosette or pill organizer. Or you can have the pharmacy put them into blister packs. This helps keep your medications organized, and you will have an easier time knowing if you have taken your medication and when the next dose is due. (These are also beneficial tools for caregivers who help others with their pills.)

Geriatricians and Specialists

If you are older than 65 and you are experiencing complicated health issues, you may want to get a referral for consultation with a geriatrician. A geriatrician is a primary care doctor who specializes in the care of older adults. Where there are a variety of specialists (e.g., for heart disease, cancer, diabetes), you will want to have one healthcare professional overseeing all of your medications, dietary needs, and treatments. Family doctors are often the natural choice, however, in some cases, you may want to seek help from someone who has specialized training. For example, in Manitoba, we have an education program out of the University of Manitoba called "Care of the Elderly," which is an enhanced-skills program for managing complex geriatric care. You may want to seek out a specialist who can manage all of the issues. Pharmacists, especially those familiar with geriatrics, can help with reviewing the medications and any interactions or contraindications. For access to a geriatric specialist, please speak with your primary healthcare professional to see if you qualify and if a referral is recommended.

Disease

Unfortunately, advanced age is a significant risk factor for many common diseases. In my clinical work, I have seen many older people who have had (or have) cancer, heart disease, heart attacks, strokes, type 2 diabetes, high cholesterol, high blood pressure, dementia, Parkinson's disease, or arthritis. Sometimes our genetic disposition or gender also adds to our risks. There are specialists who will work with you to determine the right approach to helping keep you healthy and functioning.

It is possible to live well and long with chronic diseases such as cancer, heart disease, hypertension, and diabetes. Getting symptoms checked out, such as swelling in your feet and ankles (edema), is essential, as there are many reasons for it. Following your healthcare team's advice will help you thrive despite your challenges.

Dementia (Major Neurocognitive Disorder)

Dementia is a syndrome that affects a person's memory, speech, thinking, judgement, and coordination. I did a small, informal survey and asked people what they fear more—Alzheimer's disease (A.D.) or dying. The response was unanimous—people fear getting A.D. more than death itself. Alzheimer's disease is a progressive and fatal condition of unknown cause that affects the brain and is the leading type of dementia. Other types of dementia include Vascular Dementia, Lewy Body Dementia, Parkinson's Disease Dementia, Frontotemporal Dementia, and many others. Scientific research is teaching us that there is a link between diet and dementia. If you are concerned about getting dementia or feel you are at risk, you may want to talk to your doctor or dietician about what you can do to reduce your chances.

Vision and Hearing

Two common things that happen to us as we age are a change in our vision and in our hearing. Most of us will experience some changes in our near vision around

Ultraviolet (UV) protection for your eyes matters. Choose sunglasses that protect your eyes from the potential harm done by the UVA and UVB rays of the sun.

age fifty. An eye exam will help rule out cataracts or glaucoma (if you have any serious eye conditions, you may have to see an ophthalmologist). An optometrist can check your vision, and you can get a prescription for reading glasses. You could probably get away with buying the cheaper "Cheaters" or "Reading Glasses" you find at the local discount or drug store. I can always tell when a person is too vain to get reading glasses. They are the ones squinting to read the menu or asking someone else to order for them. There is no shame in needing reading glasses. It happens to almost all of us.

The second thing that happens is we often start to lose our ability to hear well. I don't know if I have seen any older adults who *don't* have a hearing impairment. Sometimes there is a buildup of earwax that can be cleaned out. Other times a visit to an audiologist or to an ear, nose, throat (ENT) physician is needed. If there are hearing concerns, a trip to a hearing centre is an option. Many offer free hearing tests.

When I was 54, my husband said I had a hearing problem. I didn't think so. I thought perhaps he wasn't standing close enough to me, or he was mumbling. Sometimes he would talk to me from another room when I was washing dishes and listening to music—I couldn't hear him. The hearing test revealed my hearing was within normal limits, and the concern my husband had was laid to rest. A registered audiologist wrote a note saying I had, "Normal hearing sensitivity bilaterally. Recommend reducing the distance from the person speaking and the source of background noise to improve the audibility of conversation."

Sometimes a hearing aid or two is recommended. You really do get what you pay for, so, depending on your budget, try to get the best quality you can afford. New technology is always coming out, and the latest I have heard of is a Bluetooth hearing aid. There are other alternatives such as amplifiers, which work well for people who may have cognitive impairment or find it difficult to manage and manipulate hearing aids. Research has shown that older people with hearing problems have a higher risk for developing dementia. So, it's important to get used to those hearing aids sooner rather than later, as it could help prevent cognitive decline. Plus, you will have fewer chances of feeling like you are being left out if you can hear what's going on. Lip reading can get you only so far!

Disability and Frailty

Arthritis, falls, old injuries, neurological conditions, and vertigo (dizziness) can all cause problems with mobility and daily functioning. For example, a woman with arthritis in her knees can experience a lot of pain, and she may have to use a cane or walker to help her get around safely. Pain management becomes critical, especially if the pain is long-lasting. Those with balance issues may need to use a walker or hold onto someone, so they don't fall. Wheelchairs are also helpful if someone cannot walk safely due to limited strength, fall risk, or paralysis. A person who has limited range of motion in their shoulders may not be able to get a dish from the top of the cupboard. Arthritic fingers can make it difficult to open a medicine bottle. There are ways to get around these physical limitations, and if you need someone to help you do it, there is always that, too. Maybe you have to rearrange your cupboards or home. Accommodating your limitations will help you cope and manage better.

Falls and Fracture Prevention

Women are more prone to bone-density issues (osteoporosis) due to estrogen loss during menopause. Osteoporosis can cause brittle and weak bones, so it is important to be careful and avoid falls. Falls can cause broken bones, which can impair mobility and function.

I have met one too many older adults who have fallen, nearly fallen, or are afraid of taking a tumble. There are many risk factors, and it is usually a "perfect storm" that results in a fall. Preventing slips and trips is possible if you take some precautions and are mindful of some of the hazards or underlying problems that can increase your risk.

The following issues are related to falls:

1. Falling in or around the tub or shower (Solutions: Get someone to help you, install grab bars, get a bath chair and handheld shower nozzle, install non-slip mats in the tub and just outside the tub, or go big and get a walk-in bathtub)

2. Frailty (legs aren't strong, due to inactivity or neurological problems)

3. Medications that are sedating (some antipsychotics, "sleeping pills," and many others)

4. Postural hypotension (a fancy name for a drop in blood pressure upon rising, which makes one dizzy)

5. Dizziness due to vertigo, a neurological problem, dehydration, or other medical problems such as low blood sugar or low iron levels

6. Bed-to-floor falls may occur when you try to get out of bed or try to roll over. Consider a floor-to-ceiling pole, adjustable hospital bed, or bed-assist rail. Some nursing homes put up two bed rails or "crash mats" beside the bed

7. Tripping hazards—pets, leashes, cords, area rugs, purse handles, shoes, slippers

8. Falling when trying to get out of a reclining chair (consider an electric lift chair)

9. Stairs (adjust your environment so you don't have to go up or down stairs, or install a stairlift)

10. Icy or snowy conditions

11. Improper footwear

Older women are at particular risk of broken bones due to their higher rates of osteoporosis. Hip fractures can occur spontaneously in older people, but they are often the result of a fall. There are treatments for osteoporosis, so it is wise to discuss this issue with your healthcare professional. Hip protectors (special undergarments with padding to protect the hips) can be used if there are concerns about falls and breaking a hip. (As mentioned earlier, a DEXA scan can check for issues with bone density.) Osteoporosis Canada is a great resource for education, empowerment, and support (osteoporosis.ca).

To help reduce your risk for a fall, consider doing some exercises to keep you strong and limber. Balance issues can be helped with "standing on one leg" exercises. Mobility issues in the ankles can be improved by doing chair exercises such as the "Ankle Alphabet," which can be described as drawing the alphabet in the air with your toes and moving your ankles in all directions. A medication review with your doctor or a pharmacist can point out what medications may be making you feel lightheaded or dizzy. The

ANKLE EXERCISES

If you are housebound, or if nature-walks are not something you take, or your mobility is already compromised, here is an excellent exercise to do while sitting in your favourite chair, knitting, or watching television. It's very simple, and it's this: rotate your ankles. An excellent challenge is to rotate each foot, one at a time, by spelling out the alphabet in capital letters. For instance, make a letter "A," then a "B," and so on. If you have never done this, by the time you get to "Z," you are going to feel it. I am sure this works for other types of alphabets besides English. As long as you move your ankles in every possible direction, you are helping activate all those muscles, tendons, and nerve endings that help keep you upright and keep you walking.

— Janice M. Bailey

reason for that faint feeling upon rising should be investigated. Perhaps you have to move more slowly or count to three before walking. Being mindful of where your pets are at all times can help prevent you from tripping over them.

The goal is to help prevent breaking a bone or twisting an ankle. Head injuries can be serious, and a concussion can have long-lasting effects. It seems to me if you are older and break a hip, there is a big chance you may not live long after that. I don't mean to be a downer, but I have seen this situation too many times. Be careful!

Fall-Prevention Tip: Always try to keep a hand free, and hold a handrail (or at least glide your hand along it) when you are going up or down stairs. Take it slow and easy. If you want to run or go faster, just make sure you are watching your step. If you need to watch your step, or if you have any coordination issues, count your steps. It will help keep you focused on your task, thereby reducing your risk for falls. (P.S. If your stairs don't have a railing, get one installed immediately!)

"Help! I've Fallen, and I Can't Get Up"

My mom told me once when she was in her early 60s, she was in the library, looking at some books on a small shelving unit. She did a deep knee bend to look at the books on the bottom shelf, and she realized she couldn't get back up because there was nothing to hold on to. The librarian came over and helped her up. My mom said to herself, "That's enough of that." So, she made sure to include leg-strengthening exercises and stretching in her fitness routine.

Falling and experiencing a long lie on the floor can be very hazardous to your health. If you are concerned that you may not be able to get up from the floor, check out the method called "Backward Chaining" (also known as Backward Training) to help you get safely up and off the floor, unassisted. You can practice the sequence of getting down on the floor and then getting back up. Each task can be broken down into smaller steps. Techniques include kneeling, crawling, and bum-walking. You can also use a chair, sofa, or stairs to help you get up. There are some excellent

31

videos online to help demonstrate the Backward Chaining technique. If you want professional guidance on this, you may want to consult a physiotherapist.

Walking Gait

If you happen to have a bad knee or hip, it may result in favouring one leg. Even if you've had surgery, you may end up limping. I have a friend who affectionately calls herself "Gimpy" because she tends to favour one side when she walks. Some 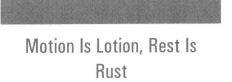 older people tend to shuffle or walk with an unbalanced gait.

Motion Is Lotion, Rest Is Rust

To help avoid falls, trips, or slips, you may want to get a physiotherapy assessment so you can get some advice on how to improve your walking. Or, perhaps you need a referral to a specialist. Knee- or hip-replacement surgery is very common in older adults who have arthritis.

A custom-made foot orthotic insert for your shoes can help improve your balance by correcting any misalignment in your foot and ankle. A podiatrist is a specialist in foot, ankle, and lower-leg problems.

Physical Activity

This isn't going to be a book all about exercise, as there are plenty of books, videos (remember the "Prancercise" lady, Cher, Jane Fonda, and Richard Simmons?), and classes you can learn from. You don't have to aspire to be a "SuperAger," but I would encourage a modest and healthy approach to staying active throughout your lifespan. I can't emphasize enough the importance of physical activity as integral in overall total wellness. (This is the longest chapter in the book, by the way!) Please also note, if you are going to consider starting any new exercise regime, discuss it with your healthcare provider first. If given the green light, consider seeking guidance from a registered physical therapist, physiotherapist, or athletic therapist for assessment and a plan of care that is safe and suited to your specific needs.

I grew up in Canada watching BodyBreak commercials with Hal and Joanne. Their "Keep fit and have fun" mantra was a regular occurrence in my day. Watching TV was a pleasurable activity—although we were learning that many TV watchers were not keeping as physically active as they should. Hal and Joanne would make staying active look enjoyable. By the way, they are still together, staying fit, and having fun.

AN ACTIVE LIFE IS A BETTER LIFE

There are many free fitness apps. The ParticipACTION app was designed to get people of all ages and abilities active. The "Everything gets better when you get active" theme provides videos, articles, encouragement, prizes (such as gift certificates), and team challenges. ParticipACTION has been encouraging Canadians to get healthy by getting active since 1971.

One time I came across a list of "100 Benefits of Exercise" posted on the wall at a gym I had joined. Soon after, I came across a list of "125 Good Reasons to Exercise" in the back of *Living the Good Life: Your Guide to Health and Success* by David Patchell-Evans. I find multiple copies of this book at thrift shops and garage sales, and I think it is one of the best generic books on exercise around. The 125 reasons start with "Exercise makes sense, because it..." and then goes on to identify all kinds of benefits to mind, body, and spirit. It's heavy on the "body" aspects and has a smattering of mind and spirit points.

Included in this extensive list are: "...increases your self-confidence and self-esteem, helps you sleep better, lifts your spirits, and helps keep you at your right body weight." It's incredible how good exercise is for you—and it's also notable that, although we all know how good it is for us, many of us don't do it. We are instinctually driven to conserve our energy and be ready for the next "big hunt." Although our lifestyles have changed (we don't need to hunt and gather for our food anymore), our inborn instincts haven't. I know I struggle with this, and I guess you may, too.

Exercise and movement are essential aspects of a well-rounded and balanced lifestyle. There are countless benefits to staying fit, and "active aging" is a term that is used a lot in the successful aging community. I believe we need to *Sweat—Strengthen—Stretch* throughout our lives, and it is even more critical as we age. The World Health Organization (WHO) recommends regular physical activity for healthy adults aged 18-64. The very minimum is 150 minutes of moderate-intensity aerobic exercise (what I call sweat!) per week. **That's about 20-25 minutes per day.** If you bump it up to more vigorous activity, you can go for 75 minutes per week. That's about 10 minutes a day. The more effort you put in, the better chance you have that your blood gets pumping through your veins and arteries, like cleaning out a clogged drainpipe. The unhealthy buildup is whisked away—much like a plumber using a strong chemical to unclog the system. Sometimes when I am exercising, I visualize a plunger cleaning out the pipes!

Not all personal trainers believe we have to sweat, though.

> We do not have to sweat during every session. Somehow, we have formed the opinion that if you did not sweat, you did not work hard enough. Not true! Exercise should not beat you up and leave you for dead on the side of the road. Not to say a good sweaty keep-fit session is not good, but it is not necessary. Exercise should energize you and make you ready to take on the world—or at least take on your day. We simply want to get the blood flowing and loosen up tight muscles and lubricate the joints.

— Donna Wieliki, Personal Trainer and Group Fitness Leader

If you want to get technical, you can look up how many "beats per minute," also known as BPM or heart rate, you need for optimal cardiovascular (heart health) benefit. Your age determines your target and maximum heart rates. Fitness trackers can help monitor your BPM. If you hire a personal trainer, they can help you develop an exercise program, including target heart rate, that will help you reach your goals.

You may even want to explore High-Intensity Interval Training (HIIT) if you like to run or cycle. You may have seen this at the gym. It incorporates bursts of high-intensity exercise for short periods of time, alternated with low-intensity recovery activity. The bursts don't have to last long (30 seconds to one minute), and you can build up your stamina to increase the duration or number of intensive boosts during your workout session.

Walk like you don't want to be late for an important meeting or appointment. This will help you pick up the pace!

Functional fitness is a term used to describe our ability to do everyday things, like get up off the floor, carry heavy items, and put something up on a shelf. Our day-to-day activities can help us keep functionally fit. We can even count some of these short bursts of movement as HIITs. Consider washing your car. You have to use a lot of muscles to wash, scrub, hose down, etc. This is known as a "high-intensity incidental physical activity" (HIIPA), according to a September 2019 editorial in the *British Journal of Sports Medicine*.

The WHO also recommends muscle-strengthening activities (what I call strengthen!) at least two days per week. The stretch part is what I may also call a cool-down or yoga. The WHO states, "Adding gentle stretching may also be beneficial." I believe flexibility is critical, and we know the more we stretch and push our limits, the more flexible we can be. For example, what if you were trying to bend down and tie your shoes, but you didn't have the flexibility to do so? Keeping limber will help you maintain your independence longer and help prevent injuries.

Speaking of injuries, there is always a risk of falling or getting hurt when engaging in any physical activity. Case in point: My husband and I decided to take out our 31-year-old cross-country skis. I lost control as I was going down a small hill. Down I went, falling backward, and I landed on my left wrist. Nothing serious, but it could have been worse. Be careful out there!

For those 65 and older, the WHO recommends the same amount of exercise as younger adults, with an additional emphasis on "functional balance and strength training." Strengthening the muscles used for balance will help prevent falls, fractures, and other related injuries.

What kinds of activities should you do? Keep in mind that the WHO states that doing *some* physical activity (*any* activity) is better than doing *none*. More than some is better.

Walking is one of the most common forms of exercise. Having proper footwear for longer walks is imperative. Hiking poles or walking sticks are also recommended in any weather or type of terrain to help keep you stabilized and work your upper body muscles (you may also need a backpack). For warmer weather, you want to make sure your feet aren't too hot, and, for colder weather, you want to have warm shoes or boots. I bought a new pair of waterproof hiking shoes that will work in almost any kind of terrain or weather. For winter, I have a pair of warm waterproof boots that are good for use on snow and slippery ice. You may want to consider getting slip-on ice cleats or traction devices that affix to your shoe or boot to help your grip on the snow and ice.

Scheduled group exercises work for some people. A gym membership can help motivate people to get moving. Some elite gyms pride themselves on having fancy group-exercise classes. The Spin Classes (indoor group cycling on stationary bikes) look pretty intense with the music, lights, and the instructor yelling out and encouraging people to "Go hard!" I've tried a few different group classes: Zumba, Drumming, Water Zumba, Anti-gravity Fitness. Yes, I tried aerial yoga, and it was quite interesting; I felt like I was swinging on a hammock! Then there is yoga, either hot or regular. There are many different types and levels of yoga, including "restorative," which is the most gentle. The hot yoga helped me stretch and strengthen, and the "sweat" part made me feel like I was in a tropical zone. My menopausal self was glad when it was over!

Home gyms also work, but you have to be committed to scheduling your workouts into your calendar (or else the dreaded "I can do it tomorrow" excuse pops up). This also applies to going out of the house to a fitness facility. There are many different equipment options for a home gym, such as elliptical, stationary bike, treadmill, exercise ball, free weights, yoga mat, resistance bands. You may prefer not to use any equipment and rely specifically on your body weight—this is called "calisthenics." Pushups, crunches, and squats are popular strengthening calisthenic exercises. Some people call these their "floor exercises."

If you are trying to lose a few pounds, keep in mind the 80/20 rule. Weight loss occurs at a faster rate when you put more emphasis on reducing your caloric intake. It's easier to shed one pound a week by cutting out the sweets and reducing your portions rather than trying to burn more calories by increasing your physical activity. It's not *precisely* 80% diet and 20% exercise, but it's around there. Plus, drinking a big glass of water as soon as you wake up and before meals can help curb your appetite!

I like to "walk and talk" outside with a friend. We get in some exercise and some socializing at the same time. Joining a sports team to play soccer may be your idea of having fun and getting active. Learning a new dance, such as hip hop, or line dancing, can be a hoot. I took belly-dance lessons, and it was invigorating! I still have my colourful hip scarves with the jingly coins.

NO MORE LIMP

My mother has small and narrow feet. After her second hip surgery, she noticed how one foot was turning in more. She couldn't walk very straight and had a limp. She likes to travel, and it bothered her a lot when she was out sightseeing. She could feel the pain in her hips. Her doctor and physiotherapist told her there was no issue, but when she went to an Orthopedic Clinic, they discovered that one leg was shorter. A common result of hip or knee surgery is that one foot will turn in more and throw you off balance. With the proper orthopedic inserts, it has helped keep her feet 'level' and has made a huge difference. — Dana

Paddleboarding, canoeing, kayaking, or other water sports may also be a way to get out, get active, and have fun doing it. I have even tried boogie-boarding on the waves in Hawaii! That was a blast.

Parking your car in the farthest spot in the parking lot can help you get in your steps. Wearing a pedometer or using an app on your phone can help keep track of your steps. Set some goals! Challenge yourself! Don't do things the easy way—do them the *hard way*. Get up to change the TV channel versus using the remote. Ride your bike instead of driving. Do your housework instead of hiring someone to do it. Cut your lawn, shovel the snow. There are tons of ways to keep active. Get creative.

Sedentary behaviour, that is, sitting too much and having long periods of inactivity, is very unhealthy. We need to move as much as possible. Standing up and moving around for a few minutes during a commercial break is good for us. Sitting is the new smoking. Apps are available to nudge us to get up and move. The Apple watch urges us to stand up each hour. Having a pet will make us move more, too. I have a sign by my back door; it says, "Let dog in, let dog out. Let dog in, let dog out." We have two dogs, so they keep us hopping! Taking a dog for a walk also counts as exercise— for you and the dog.

If you have injuries or are dealing with medical problems that affect your mobility, you may want to see a physiotherapist or a sports therapist. They will do a personalized assessment and provide you with some exercises to try at home.

Massage Therapy

Have you ever had a back massage? Or a reflexology foot massage? There are many different types of massage, and I have certainly had my share. My first massage, in my early 20s, left me feeling battered and bruised the next day, which was completely normal, from what my therapist told me. It felt a bit awkward, as it was my first massage, but I enjoyed the feeling of the therapist's hands and fingers stretching, rubbing, and manipulating my muscles. Massage can help us relax, and it can be used in a therapeutic way to relieve tension and pain in our muscles. After a good workout, sometimes our muscles may feel sore. A good stretch can help, but a massage is even better. If you can, a monthly massage is a great way to keep the circulation moving and the muscles, joints, and ligaments in good shape. Alternatives include:

♦ A handheld massager
♦ An electric massage chair cushion
♦ Exchange massages with a friend or significant other
♦ Gently roll a ball between your back and the wall

I believe massages are good for our mind, body, and soul.

Prevention, Maintenance, and Early Detection

Immunizations against disease are recommended for folks as they age. The main ones that I am aware of are for shingles, the flu, pneumonia, and—new to the scene—COVID-19. Early-detection measures for women include:

♦ Pap tests (for cervical-cancer screening)
♦ Mammograms (for breast-cancer screening)
♦ Fecal occult blood tests and colonoscopy (for colorectal-cancer screening)
♦ Regular physical checkups at the doctor's office (frequency to be determined by your doctor)

During your complete physical exam, routine laboratory tests may include hemoglobin, white blood-cell count, red blood-cell count, thyroid, blood sugar, and additional tests, based on your health history and symptoms. Blood pressure should be checked and a physical assessment conducted, including listening to your heart and lungs with a stethoscope. The doctor may also check your eyes, mouth, ears, and lymph nodes. The abdominal exam may include listening for sounds with the stethoscope and palpating the area, feeling for lumps or discomfort.

Women should also get a manual breast exam and a digital rectal exam. Either your general practitioner or a gynecologist can help with any issues in the vaginal area. You should also see a dentist one to two times yearly for cleaning (removing the tartar buildup) and an X-ray of your teeth, as needed. If you have dentures or partials, you will want to inspect them for any breakage and make sure they fit correctly. You may need an alignment at some point. Having health insurance can help cover most of the costs of these procedures and services.

When I was 40, I had concerns about some lumps I found in my breasts. While I was doing my regular self-breast exam, I felt some very defined lumps. I was afraid of what it might be, so I made an appointment to see my doctor. I had known two other women in my workplace diagnosed with breast cancer, so I knew that having lumps could mean the worst. My doctor recommended I go for a mammogram and see a specialist. The waiting time between the mammogram and the visit to the specialist was very nerve-wracking. I've come to know this feeling as "scanxiety." The specialist took a medical history, did a manual examination, and looked at the mammogram results. She told me that what I had were "40-year-old breasts." She said that the skin tissue starts to form lumps as gravity and the years take hold. She said I didn't have to tell anyone that I had 40-year-old breasts (but I did!). At that moment, I realized my body was getting old.

To keep all your medical appointments, specialists, tests, investigations, diagnoses, and medications organized, it's vital to get a "Medical Records" organization system in place. I have a three-ring binder that I keep updated and add to as needed. Any reports I get go into my personal Medical Records binder. This also comes in handy when you see a new doctor, and they have questions for you, such as, "When was your last mammogram?" Or "What medications have you tried for this problem?"

Emergency Response Information Kit

If you are concerned about your health, you may want to consider getting an emergency-response information kit prepared. In Winnipeg, we have the E.R.I.K. program, which was developed to assist seniors, chronically ill persons, those who live alone or who have caregivers, or those who have communication or speech barriers. The complete kit contains the following information:

- Name (first, middle, last)
- Address (in full)

- Gender
- Health Card/Insurance numbers
- Family physician (name and phone number)
- First and second emergency contact people (name, phone number, and relationship)
- Medical history (include if there is heart disease, high blood pressure, diabetes, breathing problems, and other medical concerns such as illnesses and surgeries). Note: If you have a pacemaker, indicate where it is.
- Allergies and Sensitivities
- Medications—both prescription and non-prescription (name, dosage, frequency, where they are stored)
- Pharmacy (name and phone number)
- Indicate if there is an Advance Health Care Directive (i.e., Living Will) and where it is stored
- Indicate if there is an Organ Donation Card and where it is stored

You may want to include a copy of any medical-implant cards and your blood type. When completed, it is put into a plastic sleeve and attached to the fridge with a magnet. If needed, when the paramedics arrive, all of the information is available in the emergency response information kit (E.R.I.K.), which they will take to the hospital with them. More information is available, including a blank form, at winnipeg.ca/fps/Public_Education/EMS_Presentations/E.R.I.K.stm.

Stress Management

Chronic stress can lead to other health problems. Reducing stress, learning how to relax, taking time out, and perhaps slowing your mind and body down are needed to keep your hormones in check. Finding healthy ways to cope with life's stressors can help you stay healthy, and if you happen to get ill or get "knocked down" by life, it will enable you to bounce back. Building up resilience takes time and effort. Managing stress—flexing that stress-buster muscle—is necessary to help maintain physical (and emotional) well-being. More on how to manage stress in the Emotional Wellness chapter.

Self-Image and Physical Appearance

Over the years, I have observed a few things about people as we get older. One is we shrink. Whenever I ask an older adult for their height, a prevalent answer is, "Well, I've shrunk!" They usually say it in a joking manner. It seems like most of us can expect to lose an inch or two as we age, due to our shrinking spine. Osteoporosis could also be a culprit. The other noticeable change in older people is that we tend to slow down as we age. Almost everything we do is a bit slower. We walk, think, remember, speak, and move more slowly.

Depending on how we see ourselves, we could be comfortable with our appearance or be unhappy and suffer from low self-esteem. We can do many things to change our appearance (such as change our hairstyle or lose a few pounds), but there are many things we can't change. As women in this North American society, we are often judged by others in a youth-and-beauty-obsessed culture. Celebrities and top fashion models are often revered and admired for their beauty and finesse. Once they get to a "certain age," they find they are replaced with someone younger. A few celebrities have maintained their "timeless" beauty, such as Sophia Loren and Helen Mirren. Others seem to be "aging gracefully," such as Oprah Winfrey, Halle Berry, Lisa Lu, Jennifer Lopez, Susan Aglukark, Buffy Sainte-Marie, and Jennifer Aniston.

KIDS SAY THE DARNDEST THINGS

I work as a casual for a local elementary school's after-school program. Last year, a boy in grade three told me my grey was starting to show and that I needed to dye my hair...which was much funnier than the girl in grade one poking my side and saying I was "...squishy...." Good thing they are cute!

— Dana

There is a big push for us, as women, to look a certain way and "fight" the aging process. I say let's *embrace* our age and *celebrate*

> Consider a "Seasonal Colour Analysis" if you haven't done one already. Find out what colours flatter the natural tones of your skin, hair, and eyes.

who we are. The anti-ageism movement has helped us make strides towards embracing our age and all its wrinkles.

One of the biggest and most acceptable ageist things we do to ourselves is colour over our grey hair. Two of my closest friends have been colouring their dark hair for decades now. I wonder if and when they will ever decide to let their grey be free? It seems that my friends who had lighter hair to begin with (blond) have an easier time with embracing their greys. In my mid-fifties, I was about 10% grey, and I used to have a problem with it and ensure my hairdresser covered up the greys with hair dye. I am not as bothered by it anymore. I also have a Mallen streak, a strip of grey hair that I wear with pride.

We can change our look with the latest fashion trends, hairstyle, hair colour, and footwear. Jewelry and makeup can also be fun, no matter what your age. Some people say we have to be careful and "dress our age." What does that even mean? I like to shop in my closet and drawers and find things hiding or tucked away—those items I've forgot about. Wearing bright-red lipstick, colouring your hair pink, wearing a miniskirt, or doing whatever you please is totally up to you. I once read that the time you should stop wearing red lipstick is age 59 (!). Any other colour will do, I guess? Perhaps you choose to wear no makeup and wear sweatpants all the time—you don't go for the hype or pressure. Anything goes, as long as you feel good.

I have seen a few women in my clinical work who are upset with the aging process and unhappy with themselves. Certainly, we may grieve the loss of our youth, and we may feel sad that we can't do some of the things we used to do before, but hopefully, we will get over it with time.

I have two easy tips that will instantly improve your appearance. Any time you are feeling frumpy or down, do this:

1. **Straighten up!** Shoulders back, chest out, head up! And if you want, try holding in your stomach (tighten your core). We often neglect our posture, so we need to be reminded. If you need to use a cane or walker, it's essential to ensure it's the right height so you can walk without bending over. If required, consider special garments or a back brace to keep your body upright. Also, beware of "Text Neck Syndrome." Looking down at your devices all the time can cause neck and back problems. Keep your chin up!

2. **Smile!** The quickest way to make you feel and look good is to put a smile on your face. As we age, lines and crevasses form, and it may look like we have a "permafrown" (a permanent frown or sad face). A simple lift of the corners of your mouth can improve your appearance. And you don't need to go a full-on smile; just a little bit will help. The line from the corner of our lips to our chin tends to deepen and lengthen over time. The nasolabial folds, or "smile lines," those lines that go from your nose to the outside of the corner of your lips, will also become more pronounced, but heck! That's from all the smiling and laughing you will be doing. That's a good thing, right? (Try it in front of a mirror, and see what you think.)

Addiction

Alcohol use is legal in North America. It is not available to children, but sometimes they get their hands on it (especially teenagers). We see alcohol use on TV (women drinking a glass of wine or men having a beer), so it is very normalized. Smoking used to be very acceptable and normalized. However, now that we know the dangers to our health, we don't see it in popular culture as much. Alcohol can be addictive, just like smoking cigarettes. We are learning more about the effects of alcohol on our bodies. For example, brain health can be affected if we have too many drinks in a week. Alcohol use increases cancer risk. As people age, the dangers of drinking increase because of other factors such as medication interactions and increased risks of falls.

There are low-risk alcohol-usage guidelines that can help prevent adverse effects from drinking. For adults in general (18-64), the Canadian Centre on Substance Use and Addiction states that the upper limit for women should be 10 drinks a week with no more than two standard drinks a day, and, for adult men, no more than 15 drinks a week, with no more than three standard drinks a day. Keep in mind a standard drink is 12 ounces of beer with a 5% alcohol content, a 5-ounce glass of wine with a 12% alcohol content, and 1.5 ounces of the hard stuff (such as rye, gin, rum, vodka) at 40% alcohol content. For women age 65 or better, they suggest no more than one standard drink a day, with no more than five drinks per week. For men 65 and older, no more than one to two standard drinks per day with no more than seven in total. Non-drinking days are recommended for every week.

> I add some water to my small serving of red wine. My late mother-in-law used to do this (and she was Italian). It reduces the alcohol content per ounce while allowing you to enjoy the social aspects of drinking wine without getting "loopy." Our bodies can't handle liquor like it used to. Now I and many of my peers consider ourselves "lightweights."

If you feel you have a daily craving or urge to drink alcohol—and once you get started, you find it's hard to stop—you are probably addicted and may want to talk to your doctor about getting help. You may need to go into rehabilitation. The same goes for illicit drugs (e.g., heroin, crack, cocaine) and prescription pain or anxiety medication (e.g., narcotics, opioids, benzodiazepines). Addiction to substances is a medical issue (physiological dependence) that comes with a psychological component. Support groups such as Alcoholics Anonymous or other programs such as Smart Recovery can help as well. Smart Recovery can help with not only substance addictions but problem behaviour.

45

It is possible to develop an addiction to anything. This has to do with the reward pathway in the brain. In addition to dev-eloping a physiological addiction (such as nicotine), we can develop psychological addictions. Gambling —in person or online —can be financially devastating. I've heard online gambling is one of the most challenging addictions to overcome, due to its widespread availability. There is also the allure of the fun and excitement of being in a casino, which can hook some people without them even knowing it. It's not unheard of for people to get way in over their heads and end up being in debt by \$25,000 to \$40,000 or more before seeking help for their gambling addiction.

We have heard of those horror stories where people become addicted to pornography or sex. These problem behaviours can ruin lives, marriages, and families. A shopping addiction can result in crowded homes and hoarding situations. If you or someone you know has an unhealthy addiction, please get help.

Menopausal Changes

Menopause is a time in a woman's life where she has not had a menstrual period for 12 months. Perimenopause, the time before menopause, can last for years. This hormonal time in a woman's life can interrupt her activities and cause a disruption. Hot flashes, painful sex (dyspareunia) due to a dry vaginal canal, and disrupted sleep due to night sweats can all create difficulties and challenges. Some women prefer to go on hormone replacement therapy (HRT), while others prefer to "sweat it out." There are risks associated with HRT, however, if you have a family history (often, even if you don't) of breast cancer. The Mayo Clinic reports that an HRT pill (called Prempro) increased the risk of not only breast cancer but also heart attack, stroke, blood clots, dementia, and uterine cancer.

Some creams and tablets can be used inter-vaginally to help with the dryness. Lubrication during sexual intercourse can help. There isn't anything I have found that works for the night sweats other than time. Natural herbs and remedies may promise relief, but I think, in the end, it's just a waste of time. If you do end up getting any kind of relief with those alternative therapies, I would say you got very lucky with your timing—or it's the placebo effect.

Hair, Skin, Teeth, and Nails

I read a good book by Dr. Cheryl Townsend called *The Aging Gracefully Pathway: A Toolkit for the Journey*. She talked about the importance of looking after our teeth and gums. Flossing, brushing, and seeing a dentist regularly can help keep gum disease at bay and can extend our lifespan. I can't remember if she mentioned this, but one way to keep your teeth looking good is to whiten them. There are some affordable options, such as whitening strips, and some toothpastes claim to help with this.

One of the many tips I picked up from Dr. Townsend's book was, after washing your hair, don't be too rough when you towel-dry it. Be gentle with your hair, so you don't break it. I took this to heart, and I believe my hair has never been healthier. I always use a good conditioner after washing my hair (two to three times weekly) to keep it from becoming brittle and dried out. A hair masque (or mask) is also a great way to help add extra protection to aging, dry, colour-treated, or brittle hair. This thick, rich restorative cream is available usually in a single-use package or a jar. I use it every 7 to 10 days. I use a styling aid and spray-on protectant as well and am careful not to damage my hair.

Stress can make our hair fall out. Chemotherapy can do that, too. I experienced hair loss in 2017 during and after my cancer treatment. My hair thinned, and I was fearful it would all go down the drain (it didn't, thank goodness). There are different things we can do to encourage hair growth. I talked to my hairdresser, and she recommended a brand of shampoo and conditioner that was helpful. I also saw a doctor who specialized in conditions of the hair and scalp. As my stress dissipated, and I tried some different remedies, my hair eventually grew back.

The skin-care industry is enormous. As we age, our skin loses its elasticity. I do a test on the top of my hand to see how much elasticity I have. You can try it, too. Flatten out one of your hands, palm down. Gently pinch and lift a small portion of your skin with your other hand. Notice how slowly or quickly the skin goes back down. If your skin is more elastic, it will go down fast. If your skin is older and less supple, it will go back slowly. One easy and economical way to help keep our skin supple and less flaky is to moisturize it. There is no need to spend a lot of money on moisturizers. The trick is to put the cream on when your skin is still damp—for example, when you get out of the shower or after you wash your hands or face.

I don't care what any of the ads say—there is no way a "wrinkle" cream will get rid of your wrinkles. It may help reduce the appearance, but it won't make them go away. Don't get caught up in the hype. It's a waste of money. And don't forget to put cream on your neck and upper chest! I put on moisturizer every morning and night to clean damp skin. It makes my skin feel better. During the day, if you are going to be outside, consider using a skin cream that has sunscreen (SPF).

Hydration and moisturizers are a woman's best friends. Both of these things will help you feel better on the inside and outside. The more hydrated and moisturized we are, the better. Drinking water and keeping our skin and nails moisturized with lotions and oils will help us look and feel good. Dry skin is irritating! We can even use moisturizers for our eyes, mouth, and vaginal area. We tend to get dryer everywhere, especially after menopause.

Natural cleansers and moisturizers are most healthy, and I have found the following ingredients (in various products) to be best for maintaining healthy skin (your list may be different):

- Green tea
- Aloe vera
- Olive oil
- Vitamin E

There are always new ideas coming out to help keep our skin looking and feeling supple. At the time of writing this book, hyaluronic acid was all the rage.

Some other tips to consider for having healthy skin are:

1. **Wear sunscreen, and avoid too much direct sunlight**. As good as the sun is for us, it can also cause damage to our skin. It can cause premature aging and, at the worst, skin cancer. Wearing a wide-brimmed hat can protect

your scalp, ears, and face. There are all kinds of hats! I have a few, and I even have one I can wear in the water, with a tie so it won't blow off. Don't forget to use sunscreen on your hands and arms (or cover them up!), as they are very vulnerable to the harsh effects of too much sun. Ensure the sun protection factor (SPF) is high enough to protect your skin, and reapply as necessary. When we were in Costa Rica, we were told we needed an SPF of at least 30. SPF 30 is also recommended by the Canadian Cancer Society.

2.   **Exfoliate**. Dry brushing is one way to exfoliate your skin, using a long-handled brush with natural fibres. This is best done in the shower; you will see lots of dead skin fall off, and then you can shower it off and remember to put a good moisturizing cream or oil on afterward. I also use a Green Tea Scrub (by St. Ives) in the shower to exfoliate my face, neck, arms, and hands.

I have found a great tip to help keep my nails healthy and looking good. As I have aged, my nails sometimes get a little discoloured, and it's more noticeable when I have removed the nail polish (I like to treat myself with a pedicure and get my toenails painted). The nails may look dry and have some white spots on them. I found skin lotion helps keep them moisturized, however, the best thing I have found is a Vitamin E skin and nail oil. It is a clear, sticky, thick liquid (comparable to molasses or corn syrup), and it is applied with either a cotton-tipped swab or a nail-polish brush. It's a bit messy, so just be careful when you apply it!

While I'm on the topic of toenails: Our feet are happy when we take care of them. Foot soaks (or a dip in a fancy foot bath) are fun, especially when we add Epsom salts or other soothing ingredients to the water. I like to add some essential oils like peppermint and rosemary. Softening up the skin helps slough off the dead layer and makes the nails ready for trimming. If you can't cut your nails comfortably or safely, or if you have diabetes or other foot problems, you may consider getting your nails trimmed by a foot nurse or podiatrist. Calluses and warts on the feet are common issues that your healthcare provider can give you guidance on.

Physical health and well-being are determined by our genetics, our environment, and our behaviour. If we make healthier choices, follow our healthcare professionals' advice, keep active, and practice prevention, maintenance, and early detection, we can increase our chances of living healthier, happier, and longer. Do a self-assessment, and see where you can make some improvements.

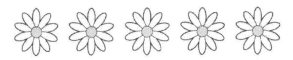

Physical Wellness Self-Assessment

On a scale of 1 to 4, 1 being very dissatisfied, 4 being very satisfied, where are you at in terms of satisfaction with your physical health?

Circle one:

1 = Very dissatisfied. Horrible. Nonexistent.
2 = Dissatisfied. Not that great.
3 = Satisfied. It's okay.
4 = Very satisfied. Very content. Happy.

Physical-Wellness Reflection

If you score on the bottom half of the scale, what can you do, moving forward, to improve your physical health score? And when do you want to start making changes? How important is this to you? If you are scoring in the top half of the scale, what can you do to move toward a "four"?

Affirmations

- I am active and healthy.
- I eat to nourish my body.
- I enjoy a personalized, balanced diet.
- I am at a healthy weight and waist circumference.
- I look after my body and practice prevention.
- My immunizations are up to date.

- I maintain my teeth and gums.
- I find time to relax and rest, as I know it's essential.

Things to Try

- Take an exercise class, either in person or online.
- Find a walking buddy, and go for regular walks.
- Try making a smoothie that includes fruits and vegetables.
- Read up on "superfoods" such as olive oil.
- Research different types of diets and meal plans, and find one that suits your lifestyle.
- Commit to improving your overall physical health.
- Book a massage.
- Download an app that can help you with your health and fitness goals (e.g., exercise, diet, yoga).

References

Buettner, Dan (2010). *The Blue Zones: Lessons for Living Longer from the People Who've Lived the Longest.* National Geographic, USA.

Carr, Allen (2016). *Allen Carr's Easy Way for Women to Quit Drinking: The original easyway method.* (Available in paperback, Kindle, audiobook.)

Carr, Allen (2018). *Allen Carr's Easy Way for Women to Quit Smoking: The bestselling quit-smoking method of all time.* (Available in paperback and Kindle.)

Diaz, K. M., Howard, V. J., Hutto, B., Colabianchi, N., Vena, J. E., Safford, M. M., Blair, S. N., and Hooker, S. P. (2017). Patterns of Sedentary Behavior and Mortality in U.S. Middle-Aged Older Adults: A National Cohort Study. *Annals of Internal Medicine,* 167(7). https://doi.org/10.7326/M17-0212. Retrieved 14 Jan 2021.

Garber, C. E., Blissmer, B., Deschenes, M. R., Franklin, B. A., Lamonte, M. J., Lee, I-M., Nieman, D. C, and Swain, D. P., American College of Sports Medicine (2011). American College of Sports Medicine position stand. Quantity and quality of exercise for developing and maintaining cardiorespiratory, musculoskeletal, and neuromotor fitness in apparently healthy adults: guidance for prescribing exercise. *Med Sci Sports Exerc.* Jul: 43(7): 1334-59. PMID: 21694556. doi: 10.1249/MSS.0b013e318213fefb. Retrieved 14 Jan 2021.

Grace, Annie (2018). *This Naked Mind: Control Alcohol, Find Freedom, Discover Happiness & Change Your Life.* (Available in paperback, Kindle, audiobook.)

Government of Canada. *Canada's Food Guide.* https://food-guide.canada.ca/en/ Retrieved 15 Feb 2021.

Lamb, Sandra (June 13, 2019). *When Thinner Isn't Better.* AARP. https://www.aarp.org/health/healthy-living/info-2019/weight-concerns-after-80/Retrieved 09 Jan 2021.

Liu, Chin-Mei & Lee, Charles Tzu-Chi (2019). "Association of Hearing Loss with Dementia." *JAMA Netw Open*, 2(7):e198112. doi:10.1001/jamanetwordopen.2019.8112. Retrieved 14 Jan 2021.

Mayo Clinic (2019). "Belly fat in women: Taking—and keeping—it off." Mayoclinic.org/healthy-lifestyle/womens-health/in-depth/belly-fat/art-20045809. Retrieved 07 Mar 2021.

Mayo Clinic (2017). "Vitamin B-12." Mayoclinic.org/drugs-supplements-vitamin-b12/art-20363663. Retrieved 14 Jan 2021.

Mayo Clinic (2020). "Vitamin D and Related Compounds (Oral Route, Parenteral Route)." Mayoclinic.org/drugs-supplements /vitamin-d-and-related-compounds-oral-route-parenteral-route/description/drg-20069609. Retrieved 14 Jan 2021.

Patchell-Evans, David (2002). *Living the Good Life: Your Guide to Health and Success.*

Stamatakis, E., Johnson, N. A., Powell, L., Hamer, M., Rangul, V., and Holtermann, A. (2019). "Short and sporadic bouts in the 2018 U.S. physical activity guidelines: Is high-intensity physical activity the new HIIT?" *British Journal of Sport Medicine*, 53:1137-1139.

World Health Organization (2020). "WHO Guidelines on Physical Activity and Sedentary Behaviour." (Free .pdf report available for download from who.int.)

World Health Organization (2011). "Waist circumference and waist-hip ratio: Report of a WHO expert consultation, Geneva, 8-11 December 2008. (Free .pdf report available for download from who.int.

Chapter 4

Emotional Wellness

*If I am not good to myself, how can
I expect anyone else to be good to me?*

— Maya Angelou

I have heard it said that there are only two emotions: love and fear. All others stem from these. I wish it were that easy to explain, but another way to look at it is that there are seven basic emotions: surprise, joy, sadness, anger, fear, disgust, and curiosity. There are different intensities—and volumes. We can be a little sad or absolutely devastated. If you watch movies and read fictional books full of drama, you may also recognize other types of feelings: anxiety, interest, confusion, and contempt. It would take another book to discuss them all!

No matter what your opinions are about emotions, or how many there are, the fact is that we are human, and we all experience feelings of some form or another. About 10% of the population have trouble putting feelings into words, describing, or recognizing them (a personality trait called alexithymia). The other 90% of us bump along, experiencing all kinds of physical sensations and thoughts that accompany feelings. Some of us are very dramatic and like to express our emotions very openly, and others tend to keep them to themselves.

Having emotional wellness means you have the ability to acknowledge the decisions you make and then accept the outcomes with emotional stability and positivity.

We are born with certain personality traits—some may say it's ingrained in our soul (see the Spiritual Wellness chapter). The environment, as well as how we are raised, helps shape and mold how we view and react to our world. Certain parts of our personality are encouraged, and other parts are discouraged. Our attitudes towards life and getting older is a big part of our character.

Past traumas in our childhood can affect how we react to the world. Those who experienced trauma must be careful not to take on a "victim mentality." Post-traumatic stress disorder (PTSD) is a devastating condition that can be treated. We can learn how to reframe how we see things. Psychotherapy, body-based techniques, and energy work (e.g., Reiki) can help treat trauma and other emotional problems.

An attitude of gratitude will help get you through any difficult time.

I have always viewed life with a positive attitude. It is easy for me to see the bright side of life. When it comes to developing and determining my attitudes, I have an instinctual reaction to things. My view towards hardships is that I believe life is full of ups and downs, and these difficult times make me appreciate the good times. I tend to appreciate even the smallest of joys. I am a self-proclaimed "realistic optimist," and I always "hope for the best and prepare for the worst." When I first started working in the medical field, I heard a doctor say a term that really hit home with me. My co-worker asked him if he thought there would ever be a cure for multiple sclerosis (MS). He said he was "cautiously optimistic." That's how I like to proceed through life. That's how I got through my cancer diagnosis and treatment.

Think about the people in your life, and consider their attitudes. When you think of your parents, do you think you inherited any of their personality traits? My mom's father was always a jokester and was kind to everyone. I can see how my mom picked up that personality trait. If, deep down in our soul, we have positive, kind, loving feelings, it will show through our personality. The opposite is also true.

Consider the first "emotions" expressed by babies or young children. It usually looked like sadness, fear, or discomfort. These are the only ways a baby can communicate. Is it an actual emotion at this point? A few months later, a laughing or smiling baby is highly rewarded by its parents, and they will soon learn it's far more pleasurable to be laughing and smiling based on others' reactions. Sometimes a baby or young child cries due to wanting something they can't have. A "temper tantrum" can erupt, where the emotional floodgates open, and there is crying, yelling, and thrashing about. As young children grow up, they learn through guidance and discipline how to appropriately express emotions through talking it out and putting a name to the feelings experienced.

As we get older, some of us repress those felt emotions, and it becomes problematic due to the "bottling up" of feelings. Sometimes I use the analogy of a "pressure cooker." Emotions can get caught up in the tightly closed and locked pressure cooker. You may become angry at something that happened, but you don't express it, so it stays inside the pressure cooker. Slowly, the pressure, stress, and emotions build up. The lid is on (the emotional floodgate), but it starts to loosen up due to the buildup. Then something that seems insignificant causes another upset, and this time, "BOOM!" the lid blows off, expelling with it all the emotions that have been holed up in the pressure cooker. This catastrophic event can cause harmful and irreparable damage to relationships, especially if things are said that weren't meant to be said. Letting off the pressure or the steam can feel good, but at what cost?

Keeping a journal will change your life
in ways you'd never imagined.

— Oprah Winfrey

We can learn how to express emotion in a more appropriate, safe, and less harmful way. Communication skills can make it easier to say how you feel. Journaling or writing down your feelings can also help. Putting a pen in your hand and writing down your thoughts can help you express your emotions in a safe and nonjudgmental way. Talking to a trusted friend, family member, or a counselor can also help. Some people find comfort in joining groups or reading self-help books on subjects that are troubling to them. Education and learning about ourselves can be very enlightening. Self-awareness is often the desired outcome, with many benefits.

Stress is a part of our everyday lives. Some stress can be good, but chronic stress can be harmful. We can have too much—or not enough (bored). If we are struggling at work, home, or in our family or social circles, we have to learn how to cope with stress in a way that is healthy.

Unhealthy coping mechanisms include smoking, alcohol, drugs, gambling, emotional eating, or other unhealthy habits. Habits can turn into cravings, which can turn into addictions, so I would advise you to be familiar with low-risk guidelines. If you find yourself experiencing problem drinking, gambling, or drug use, please seek help from an addictions specialist. Healthy stress-management strategies include deep breathing, mindfulness-based stress reduction, meditation, and exercise (including yoga).

Self-esteem is at the root of how we feel about ourselves. Do you love yourself? Have you ever thought about how you treat yourself? People who have low self-esteem often feel depressed. Sometimes our feelings towards ourselves are rooted in the way we were raised. Our upbringing influences our personalities. If we were treated well and were taught self-love, then we have a better chance of having a healthy sense of self.

A related concept is self-image. If you love yourself, then you may have a healthy sense of your self-image. Knowing how you present to the world and being aware of what you want others to see reflect a healthy sense of self-esteem and self-image (more on self-image in the Physical Wellness chapter). If you don't care about yourself or how you present to the world, you may want to talk to someone to see if this can be explored and improved. Maya Angelou once said, "The real difficulty is to overcome how you think about yourself."

Forgiveness towards others and even ourselves is difficult. It may seem like an admission of weakness or error—which is an insult to our ego. People, including ourselves, will make mistakes. Telling someone you are sorry, accepting the apology, and letting go of past wrongdoings goes a long way. Saying "Sorry" to our self is equally (if not more) important. Self-compassion is learned. It's a necessary skill to have if we want to feel contentment. Let go of regrets.

Release the "shoulda, coulda, woulda" attitude, and be free. Don't be so overly critical of yourself.

When I was a mom of young children, I remember being very busy and putting a lot on my plate. Sometimes I would feel like I couldn't handle it all. When I learned to prioritize my tasks and delegate some responsibilities, it helped immensely. Sometimes there are things we think we need to put on the top of our To-Do List, but it isn't necessary at all. Who

> Sometimes the greatest pressure we experience is that which we put upon ourselves.

cares if the dishes don't get done tonight? There's always tomorrow. So what if I didn't pick up the mail today? I can send my mom flowers for her birthday instead of buying, wrapping, and mailing a parcel. We just have to realize we can't be Superwoman and not take on too much. Our enthusiasm to help others can often leads to stress and burnout.

A common goal of many people is to be happy—the elusive "Pursuit of Happiness." Most of us are motivated to do things that make us feel good versus doing things that upset us or make us angry. As we get older, we learn how to speak up for ourselves, and we tend to have less tolerance for bullcrap (that is not a professional term, but you know what I mean, right?). We start to realize that our lives are finite (we will die one day), and we make the conscious choice to live a happy life. Some of us are stuck on the "instant gratification treadmill" and want and desire things that we think will make us happy. However, "it" usually makes us happy for only one day. The excitement and anticipation of something is half (or even more than half) the fun! Being happy and content with what we have—versus what we want—is the bigger challenge.

The good news is, it is generally believed that, as we age, we tend to get happier. Although research studies are mixed, it is safe to say that we are happiest at the beginning of our lives and towards the end of our lives. It's called the U-shaped "happiness curve" of life (check out the work of Blanchflower and Oswald from 2004). Unfortunately, many people tend to experience increased anxiety and panic during midlife. Isn't this a perfect backdrop for a midlife crisis? The working years can be stressful. Luckily, we tend to experience a good sense of well-being and life satisfaction as we get older. In fact, a detailed analysis of subjective well-being that came out of the UK in 2019 finds that that people are happiest at ages 16 and 70.

For some, though, mental-health problems such as depression or anxiety may be an issue. It is not normal to feel depressed as we age. Often we confuse grief and loneliness with depression. We endure many losses in a lifetime. We lose friends and family members due to illness, moving away, death, and other reasons. Sometimes we end up going our separate ways. At times, family members (or friends) become estranged (they become strangers to us, and we don't speak to them anymore). It can be mutual or one-sided. We can experience loss of function—such as a loss in our ability to walk safely, or we may forget to take our medications. Some people have to move or downsize, which causes a loss in our familiar environment and our personal possessions.

You may benefit from seeking guidance or a professional assessment if you feel depressed or anxious. There are many helpers that you can choose from: social workers, psychologists, psychiatrists, general practitioners, and nurse practitioners. Professionals can help determine the best options to help you cope with your low mood or anxiety. Keep in mind that some people struggle with lifelong anxiety. I have seen many older adults who have dealt with anxiety all their life. It can also be part of one's personality, and it may never go away. Perhaps you are trying to learn how to cope with it. Cognitive behavioural therapy (CBT) combined with medication is one of the most effective treatments for depression and anxiety.

Left unchecked, clinical depression can lead to functional problems such as memory decline, self-neglect, isolation, or poor nutrition. It can even lead to suicidal thoughts or actions. Make sure you talk to a healthcare professional if you notice any of these concerns in yourself or a loved one.

Cognitive behavioural therapy (CBT) can be a life-changer. It's based on the premise that our thoughts, what our brain and "soul" think about, cause us to have feelings. In turn, these feelings cause us to react or behave in a way that can be either productive and healthy or unhealthy and disruptive. Some emotions come with physical reactions. We may tremble when we are scared or anxious. We may cry if we are overjoyed. Our face may flush if we are embarrassed. Learning about our thoughts and how they affect us emotionally can help us become more aware of our assumptions. It is believed that our thoughts are more easily controlled than our emotions.

STRESS BUSTER

This mindfulness exercise will help you "get out of your head."

If you feel stressed, anxious, panicky, or overwhelmed, you can try the "5-4-3-2-1 Grounding Technique." You may have heard the term "Monkey Mind." 5-4-3-2-1 helps us focus on our five senses, bringing awareness to our surroundings and the present moment. Try it now. Look for five things you can see, four things you can feel, three things you can hear, two things you can smell, and one thing you can taste. Sit with it for a couple of minutes. ❀

SITUATION → THOUGHTS → FEELINGS → PHYSICAL REACTION → BEHAVIOUR

Studies have shown that CBT with older people is often very effective. This type of psychotherapy includes homework (practice and self-reflection) between sessions. You can even do it online! CBT teaches us to shift our thinking, which changes how we react emotionally. We also learn that other people can't make us feel a certain way—it's our thoughts about the situation that cause our feelings.

Feelings aren't good or bad—they are all okay and part of the human experience. What we experience is often a normal reaction to an abnormal or new situation. If chronic and unhealthy, this reaction can concern ourselves or others, and it can lead to problems if it goes unchecked. Clinical depression or other mental illness can be debilitating, so if this is a concern for you, it's always a good idea to seek help from a professional.

Midlife can also cause a lot of change in the emotional department. For women, hormonal changes can cause mood swings. Some women may find the menopausal transition difficult as they realize (even subconsciously) it is the end of their childbearing years. Perimenopause (the time before menstruation stops, which could take years!) and the years after menopause can be accompanied by uncomfortable symptoms of hot flashes, disrupted sleep, or other physical discomforts. For others, menopause can offer a sense of freedom and opportunity. There may be a sense of freedom from the fear of getting pregnant and worrying about getting their period.

Men and women at midlife may decide to end relationships, buy new cars, change jobs, or do something else drastic due to the realization that life is finite (thus, the term "Midlife Crisis"). The realization that they are mortal beings suddenly becomes very real, and they don't want to wait to be happy or miss out on experiences they have always wanted to do. Some realize they have more years behind them than they have ahead of them, and the "clock is ticking." Conversely, some sail through without noticing anything. When people get into their 70s and 80s, they may feel time pressure. I have heard my dad, at age 75, say, "There is so much to do, and I don't have forever. I am so busy!"

A few years back, I decided to cut back on the news. Watching the news on television can be very upsetting. Rarely is there ever good news. I found myself feeling burdened with all the heaviness. Mass shootings, terrorist attacks, wars, political unrest, pandemics, natural disasters, and other unpleasant incidents were filling my head and heart. I decided to reduce my news consumption drastically, and it helped my frame of mind. I am keeping up with global and local events by reading a few headlines during the day. I have found myself happier and more intolerant of society's fixation on others' suffering. Watching too much news "desensitizes" us in some ways. I guess, for some people, it "puts their lives into perspective." I am not really sure why, but I know watching too much news is not good for me. If there is something that will affect my family or me directly, I am sure I will hear about it.

Take notice of how you feel after watching the news. If it brings you down or causes you to feel unsettled in some way, consider reducing your habits, and see if it helps. Try watching a different channel or site. Watching the news may have an opposite effect on you and help you feel more relaxed, knowing there are things going on that you may not have otherwise known about (e.g., improvements to the environment).

When we create peace, harmony,
and balance in our minds,
we will find it in our lives.

— Louise Hay

Instead of watching the news before bed (which will most likely put negative images and stories in your head), consider reading a good book, doing crosswords, listening to music, or snuggling with a cuddle buddy. If you use an electronic device such as a smartphone or a tablet, make sure you give yourself some screen-free time right before you fall asleep. The blue light (think bright blue sky on a sunny day!) that comes off the screens can trick our bodies into thinking it's still daytime, making it harder to fall asleep.

Speaking of light, I have learned that my mood and energy can be lifted if I give myself some "light therapy" daily. Sit in front of a sunny window for about twenty minutes, or go outside. Just make sure the light gets into your eyes, indirectly. The longer, the better, of course. That's why I feel better at the office, with big windows that allow light in, versus my dark, dingy computer room at home that has hardly any natural light coming in. There are light-therapy lamps available for purchase, but I haven't purchased one yet. I have heard people use them to help treat Seasonal Affect Disorder (SAD). SAD can affect people more in the winter months due to the decrease in natural sunlight caused by shorter days and the tendency to stay indoors because of the cold weather.

One day in February, I was sitting outside, getting some natural light. It was -3 degrees Celsius (27 degrees Fahrenheit), cold, but not windy. The sunlight was filtered through the clouds. A couple blocks away, I heard children playing outside in the schoolyard. It made me think. Children are generally happy and carefree. Is it the "forced" time outdoors in the natural light that helps keep them vibrant and energized? Maybe adults should be forced outdoors daily, too. We can learn from nature. Plants like to be near the sun. Dogs and cats tend to find sunny spots to lie in. Natural light is good and can help us thrive.

Practicing gratitude is another way to help improve your mood. When I was a working mom with young children, I started to feel overwhelmed and found I was losing touch with myself. I was beginning to focus on the negative aspects of my life. I was having coffee (actually, I drink tea) with a good friend, Maureen, one day, and she asked me if I have ever tried writing a "Joy Journal." I had not, so she told me more about it. There are many things you can do with a personal journal.

The first thing I did was buy myself a beautiful journal and start writing down all the things that brought me joy. I kept adding to that list until I was completely in touch with myself. Then daily, I wrote down three things I was grateful for. I did this right before bed. They were simple things, such as, "I am grateful for my house" and "I am grateful it was a beautiful sunny day." I started focusing on all the good things in my life and the things I was appreciative of. It turned my attitude and thinking around, and I was very grateful for my friend's idea. I treasure my Joy Journal, which I like to look back at once in a while to remind me of what brings me joy.

> *River rafting and mud sliding are a lot of fun, and the latter is very messy. Wear what you are willing to throw away.* — Dana

Having fun and laughing is also essential. When we were kids, it seemed so easy to find something that was fun and made us laugh. As we grow older, those opportunities are harder to find. I have made a conscious effort to seek fun times and laugh as much as I can. I have always been a serious person, so it does take some effort. I notice when I have something fun to look forward to, it lifts my spirits. I have participated in and organized many events that add some fun factor to my life. And as Miriam Castilla says, it's good to have at least one "Crazy-shit friend" to do stuff with. I have enjoyed a few zip lines, a

64

"60-foot drop," and pole-dance lessons, and I am always looking for more opportunities. Send ideas my way!

There are many things that can make a person smile or feel better. I love to watch funny movies and comedy shows (on TV or live.) I enjoy writers like Loretta LaRoche and Sophie Kinsella. Loretta is an internationally renowned American author and stress-management consultant who has had me laughing for years. Sophie is an English novelist who is best-known for the *Shopaholic* series.

I enjoy spending time with little children, as they can provide hours of entertainment and encourage me to play make-believe. They help me reawaken the "child within." Playing dress-ups was and will always be fun. Pets can also do the same thing. My son's cats are entertaining, as they do silly things and are always cute in photos. I have had many dogs over the years, and the most exciting time is when they are puppies. They provide much entertainment and companionship in the long run. "Pet Therapy" is good for the soul.

Ways to bring fun and laughter into your life include:

> **FUN AND GAMES**
>
> *The reason I do casual work in my retirement is for the fun, with co-workers and groups of children who love you to join in on the games. I have a new appreciation for any type of dodgeball game. The children laugh as 12 to 15 of them are pummelling me, and we all laugh as I attempt to get them. I have a very crappy aim!   — Dana*

- Laughter Yoga class
- Watching comedians
- Watching funny movies
- Get dressed up for Halloween
- Reading funny books
- Playing with children
- Sharing and reading funny jokes and sayings on the Internet
- Joining a social group

Emotional well-being is the opposite of feeling numb and dull or feeling stuck in a negative, stressful state. Life is full of ups and downs, and those down times are necessary, as they help us appreciate and experience the positive times fully. Sharing our good times with others is also a wonderful experience. Hopefully, we have those special people in our lives that will celebrate, cry, laugh, and share with us.

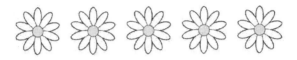

Emotional-Wellness Self-Assessment

On a scale of 1 to 4, 1 being very dissatisfied, 4 being very satisfied, where are you at in terms of satisfaction with your emotional health?

Circle one:

1 = Very dissatisfied. Horrible. Nonexistent.
2 = Dissatisfied. Not that great.
3 = Satisfied. It's okay.
4 = Very satisfied. Very content. Happy.

Emotional-Wellness Reflection

If you score on the bottom half of the scale, what can you do, moving forward, to improve your emotional health score? And when do you want to start making changes? How important is this to you? If you are scoring in the top half of the scale, what can you do to move toward a "four"?

Affirmations

- I love myself.
- I am becoming more aware of my thoughts.
- My thoughts affect my feelings, and I am working on improving my thoughts.
- My feelings aren't good or bad; they are all okay.

- These feelings will pass.
- I am considering Cognitive Behavioural Therapy and or medication to help with my struggles.
- I will seek humour and laughter more often.
- I seek joy every day.
- I look forward to being challenged by new opportunities.
- I am grateful for what I have.
- I will seek comfort and companionship from pets.
- I am sad and grieving, and that's okay.
- I am going through a midlife transition, and I will be kind to myself.
- I am pleased with what I have.
- I love the people in my life.
- I feel valued.
- I am content with my life.

Things to Try

- Look in the mirror and say "I love you" to yourself. Say it every day. Say it, and mean it. Smile. Look into your eyes.
- Write down all the things you like to do for fun to generate some ideas.
- Forgive yourself for past mistakes.
- Cut back on the news. Fill your time doing a hobby or other relaxing activity.
- If you happen to read the newspaper, skip to the comics!
- Ask your friends for recommendations of funny movies or comedians.
- Watch or record your favourite comedy movie or series.
- Share funny videos with your friends.
- Write down your thoughts and feelings in a journal.
- Honour and reflect on your midlife transition by jotting down the changes you have been through.
- Reflect on how satisfied you are with your life as a whole over the last three days.
- Call the funniest person you know.
- Watch a romantic comedy for some love, romance, and humour.
- Start a Joy Journal, and every night, write down three things you are thankful or grateful for.

- If you feel anxious, panicky, stressed, or overwhelmed, try the 5-4-3-2-1 grounding technique.
- If you are struggling with your feelings, consider seeing a therapist.
- Download an app that can help you with your goals (e.g., meditation, mindfulness)

References

Blanchflower, David G. and Andrew J. Oswald (2004). "Well-being over time in Britain and USA." *Journal of Public Economics*, 88:7-8, July 2004, pp 1359-1386.

Resolution Foundation (2019). "Happy Now? Lessons for economic policy makers from a focus on subjective well-being." Resolutionfoundation.org/publications/happy-now-lessons-for-economic-policy-makers-from-a-focus-on-subjective-well-being/ Retrieved 08 Mar 2021.

Strout, K. A., and Howard, E. P. (2015). "Five Dimensions of Wellness and Predictor of Cognitive Health Protection in Community-Dwelling Older Adults. A Historical COLLAGE Cohort Study." *Journal of Holistic Nursing* 33(1), 6-18.

Chapter 5

Brain Wellness

The key to a healthy life is having a healthy mind.

— Richard Davidson

We are born entirely dependent on others due to our underdeveloped brain. We are designed that way because of human anatomy and the birthing process. We are helpless little beings until our brains mature and we become smart enough (and strong enough) to look after ourselves. For many of us, this level of intellectual maturity (and puberty) doesn't happen until we are about 10 to 12 years old, later for boys. The teenage brain experiences a significant amount of growth and development, and sometimes this causes risky behaviour. Once our "crazy" teen years pass, and we are in our 20s, at some point, we settle down, and our productive years take over. We may seek further education, get a job, get married, have children, and pursue other exciting endeavours.

The brain is the powerhouse of our existence. We can't function independently if our brain is not working optimally. For example, someone who has a traumatic brain injury due to a motor-vehicle accident may require increased supervision. Or someone who has had brain surgery due to a tumour or other medical condition may lose part of their ability to think, talk, or walk. Those with a learning disorder or a mental illness such as schizophrenia will likely experience other challenges, as their thinking processes are very different from those of the general population.

Brain health includes cognition (the way we think, learn, store, and process information) and personality (the lens through which we view and interact with the world). The topic of "mental health," even the very term, can be one people shy away from, due to the stigma attached to the word "mental."

Mental well-being includes a healthy mind. The condition of our cognitive brain functioning—thinking, learning, and remembering—has a significant impact on our day-to-day lives. Someone who has a good level of mental health can think clearly, process information logically and sequentially, and retrieve data stored by utilizing short- and long-term memory. A healthy mind possesses a level of maturity and intelligence necessary to navigate life independently and safely. Think of cognitive functioning as the brain behind all your actions and thinking. If your cognitive health is not optimal, your overall well-being will be negatively affected.

Maintaining and nourishing a healthy brain are just as important as looking after our physical bodies. The brain is an organ, just like our heart and lungs, and everything we do physically affects all our organs' health. When we exercise, it helps get oxygen pumping through our veins, which helps get the oxygen to our lungs, heart, and brain. If we get fresh air and sunshine, the benefits are felt by not only our skin and lungs but also our brains. If we choose healthy foods, our brain is happier.

As noted earlier, it seems most people fear developing a disease like Alzheimer's more than they fear death itself. You may notice a person is "not as sharp as he used to be." You may notice "she is losing her math skills or quick-thinking abilities." Dementia hastens a person's death. It is a disease that is age-related, in that people who are older have a higher risk of developing it. Early-onset Alzheimer's disease strikes people who are younger than 65 years of age. Dementia (also known as major neurocognitive disorder) is a syndrome. It is the umbrella term used when referring to a number of conditions, such as Alzheimer's Disease, Lewy Body Dementia, Vascular Dementia, and many others.

There is currently no cure for dementia, and there is no one, sure way of preventing it. On the rare occasion, dementia can be short-term, due to other medical problems such as delirium, or when confusion is a side-effect of infection or even some medications. People who have had traumatic brain injuries, or concussions, have a higher chance of developing dementia later on in life. More on this later.

Reducing cardiovascular risks that can cause heart attacks and strokes can reduce the risk of developing dementia. Stroke can also cause dementia. Think of it as a heart attack in the brain. To reduce the risk of getting a stroke (or any other major health problem), you should:

- ✓ Avoid smoking.
- ✓ Eat a healthy diet.
- ✓ Limit alcohol use.
- ✓ Exercise regularly.
- ✓ Maintain healthy body weight.
- ✓ Reduce stress in your life.

If you have diabetes, high blood pressure, or high cholesterol, make sure you follow dietary and medication recommendations by your healthcare provider.

Many people wonder if Alzheimer's disease can be inherited. So far, research on the subject has not concluded that, if one of your parents has Alzheimer's disease, you will also get it. A gene called APOE-e4 is linked to an increased risk of late-onset Alzheimer's disease. Research is ongoing. Interestingly enough, I know of five sisters who all developed late-onset dementia. I also know of many other situations where more than one sibling developed dementia. I am not sure if these were Alzheimer's disease cases, but it makes me wonder if having a sibling with dementia increases your chances for developing it yourself.

Brain Disorders and Diseases

A person who has a mental-health illness or brain disorder will not thrive without proper diagnosis, treatment, and management. I have met and assessed many older people with mental-health issues, and they each presented with a unique set of circumstances, concerns, and goals for themselves. The primary mental-health problems I have worked with over the years include:

- Mild neurocognitive disorder (a new term for mild cognitive disorder)
- Alzheimer's disease with major neurocognitive disorder (new term for dementia)
- Vascular major neurocognitive disorder (also known as Vascular Dementia)
- Lewy Body Dementia
- Wernicke-Korsakoff Syndrome (generally related to alcohol-use disorder and thiamine deficiency)
- Major neurocognitive disorder with behavioural disturbance (formerly Behavioural and Psychological Symptoms of Dementia)
- Depression; Major Depressive Episode; Major Depressive Disorder
- Generalized Anxiety Disorder; Depression with Anxiety
- Delirium; Intermittent Delirium
- Delusional disorder
- Paranoid delusions
- Substance-use disorder (addiction)

Note: Depression and anxiety are explored more fully in the Emotional Wellness chapter.

Other mental-health problems that I have seen in my clinical work include schizophrenia, hallucinations, auditory hallucinations, musical ear, and Charles Bonnet Syndrome (seeing unusual things despite being blind).

Other related brain topics include attention deficit disorder (ADD), attention deficit hyperactivity disorder (ADHD), intellectual disabilities, dyslexia, and learning disabilities.

Another clinical area of mental health is assessing people who have personality disorders or traits. Those who had a challenging or difficult personality all their life could be having more difficulty coping or applying filters (holding back from saying or doing things that are not appropriate or socially acceptable) as they age due to the onset of dementia. Family members may start seeing a change in personality due to these changes. For example, a person who was narcissistic (very self-focused and ego-driven) all their life suddenly becomes hyper-focused on themselves and dismisses the needs of others. They feel very important and think they deserve special treatment. They want to be the first person to be served in the congregate dining room. They don't want to wait for their Home Care worker, who was delayed at the previous client's call. This is stressful for not only the person with the challenging personality but also for those around them.

Personality disorders can be tough to tease out. Psychiatrists, psychologists, and other mental-health professionals are excellent detectives and can make a diagnosis. There are several personality disorders and traits. We all have hints of, and varying degrees of, the characteristics to some extent. Still, when the behaviours and actions become harmful to others or affect the person's relationships, it becomes a "problem" that has to be understood and better managed by those who provide care. In the extreme sense, personality disorders can cause a problem with day-to-day functioning and distress.

In psychiatry terms, personality disorders are divided into three different "clusters" with three distinct personality-type quirks. Most of the personality disorders are annoying and frustrating for others. Sometimes it can get dangerous if behaviour is acted out (e.g., antisocial personality disorder).

1. Cluster A is odd or eccentric thinking or behaviour. This includes schizotypal, schizoid, or paranoid personality disorder.

2. Cluster B is dramatic or overly emotional, and unpredictable thinking or behaviour. This includes histrionic, narcissistic, borderline, or antisocial personality disorder.

3. Cluster C is anxious or fearful thinking and behaviour. This includes dependent, obsessive-compulsive, and avoidant personality disorder.

Typical personality "defects" and "quirks" include:

♦ Narcissism. "I am more important than everyone else." "What can you do for me?" "Do you know who you are talking to?" "

♦ Dependency. "I need you all the time." "I can't do anything. Please help me."

♦ Manipulation. "If you loved me, you would stay." "That other lady helped me; why aren't you helping me?"

♦ Help-seeking—Help-rejecting. "I need help. What can be done? ... No. I didn't try what you suggested. I can't do that. That won't work. I tried that already."

Personality challenges can often be overcome with cognitive-behavioural therapy and the loving kindness of others. Limit and boundary setting, patience, and understanding from others can also help in these situations.

Our personality also includes our attitudes towards things. If you have a good attitude towards aging and growing older, you will most likely be more resilient and accommodating towards any changes or upsets that come your way. If you have a negative attitude towards aging, you will probably have difficulty with it.

> **PERSONALITY QUIZ**
>
> For fun, check out the "16 Personalities" website. There you will find out what kind of "personality" you have by doing a free online test. I was an "ENFJ" last time I checked, in case you were wondering.

Trauma

There has been a lot of research done lately on the effect of trauma on people. We are all exposed to "not so nice" things in our lives, and it can have untoward lasting effects on how we move through life. Post-traumatic stress disorder can cause flashbacks and avoidance of certain situations. For example, if you experienced child abuse, you may have flashbacks at night when you are trying to sleep. Sleep is disrupted, and then you can't function properly during the day. The colonization of Indigenous people caused a lot of trauma by taking away their language and their culture. This may affect how people who are Indigenous view their world. It may prevent them from trusting specific populations again. Those who have survived a war or the Holocaust will probably carry disturbing memories of their experiences.

Traumatic injuries to the head can cause problems with thinking, learning, and processing information (think men who were boxers and fought for a living). I have heard of many people in my life who have had traumatic brain injuries or concussions. Some have trouble with vision or feel a bit confused. Kids in sports who get a concussion are often told to take a break from sports while their brain heals. Our brain is a vital organ (like most of our organs!), and it has to be protected. That's why we should wear seatbelts in the car and helmets for high-risk activities.

A stroke (a heart attack in the brain) can also cause temporary or permanent damage to your brain. Some people fully recover, while others may have memory impairment, speech impairment, or problems using one side of their body (e.g., weakness or paralysis). There are also different kinds of strokes, such as a TIA (transient ischemic attack), which is a small stroke, and there is also a silent stroke. A cerebral vascular accident (CVA) is very serious and can even lead to death.

There are many other kinds of brain injuries or illnesses that can occur, so it is always a good idea to see a doctor if there is any change to your thinking, learning, personality, or memory.

Keeping Your Brain Healthy

If you are wondering what you can do to keep your brain healthy, there are several things to do to keep it happy and flourishing. I often think of that saying, "If you don't use it, you lose it." Sitting in front of the television or scrolling on a computer screen is probably the very worst thing you could do for your brain.

Although I like to kick back and watch a television program every now and then, I realize how passive this activity is. Ultimately, I am being entertained, and I am not engaging. I also notice how easy it is to fall asleep. Do you watch television, or does your television watch you? I know someone who has a nightly ritual of lying down on the couch and "watching" television. I think he falls asleep 90% of the time. Sometimes I wonder if watching television has become the way to relax and de-stress for most people, versus being a primary entertainment source.

> **MULTITASKING**
>
> *My husband laughs at me. I love to watch TV & movies with him, but only if I have a puzzle, Scrabble on my tablet, knitting/crochet, or something else to do as I watch.* — Dana

The internet has made it so much easier for us to seek out topics of interest that engage us and at the same time provide us with social interaction on the various social-media sites. Somehow regular cable television has started to lose its appeal for some of us (perhaps it's all the commercials?). There are still many who enjoy television and the routine it offers—especially local news, sports, nature, and game shows. I watched a daytime soap opera for many years, and it was my "company" when I lived alone. The internet has also brought us the magic of being able to choose programming on our own time, suitable to our own tastes (such as Netflix or Prime Video). Social media (such as Facebook or Instagram) offer entertainment and a way to engage socially with others at the same time. There is more on social connections ahead, in the Social Wellness chapter.

People often ask me what they can do to avoid developing dementia and improve their memory skills. Although there are no guarantees, there are some things you can do to help keep your brain healthy.

How to Keep Your Brain Healthy

1. **Lifelong learning will help keep your mind engaged and active.** Take a course, learn a new musical instrument such as piano, learn to tango, or challenge yourself to learn a new language. Challenge your hand-eye coordination, and try brushing your teeth with your non-dominant hand. Take a different route to work or the shopping mall. There are lots of free courses offered on the internet and at local libraries. There is sometimes an

option where you sign up to "audit" the course. I have taken free courses on dementia, and I found them to be excellent. There are tons of YouTube videos, and you can get lost in information. Just make sure who you are learning from is reputable and not a quack or charlatan! Paid courses often offer more reputable and professional content.

2. **Play games that keep your memory skills active.** Cards, board games like Scrabble, and computer games all help stretch your memory and language skills. There are new computer games and applications (apps) for your mobile devices coming onto the market all the time. Search for terms like "brain training," "brain gym," "brain games" or "brain exercises" to see what computer programs or apps are currently available. I have seen many older people doing word-search puzzles, as they are enjoyable and help keep the brain active. Crossword puzzles and word searches are fun, too.

3. **Reminiscence helps keep old memories alive.** Looking through old photographs, gathering with friends from long ago to talk about the old days, and discussion groups can help retrieve stored memories. Often the memories are stored in our brains, but we can't retrieve them until someone cues us—then, voila! Oodles of memories appear.

4. **Physical activities that include a focus on breathing and self-awareness, such as Yoga and Tai Chi, are also very useful in keeping the brain healthy.** They can also help reduce stress and create a peaceful feeling.

5. **Mindfulness is a practice that helps you focus on the present moment.** It discourages one from thinking about the past or the future. It offers a sense of contentment as it prevents one from agonizing or worrying about past events or anxiously anticipating the future.

6.   **Meditation also helps you relax and focus on the present.** Regular practice can clear your mind and help you think straight.

7.   **A healthy diet rich in colourful vegetables and fruits, whole grains, legumes, fish, and olive oil can help reduce your chances of developing dementia (e.g., Mediterranean Diet, DASH, MIND diet, explained in more detail in the Physical Wellness chapter).**

Five Strategies to Help Improve Memory Skills

If you notice your memory skills are not as sharp as they used to be, you are not alone. Although it's not normal or inevitable, many people develop short-term memory impairment (regarding recent events).

Aging brings a variety of changes to the body. Our brain is also affected. Medications or illnesses can also cause memory problems. Dementia (impaired brain functions such as memory, speech, and planning) is also age-related, and mild cognitive impairment can be a precursor to Alzheimer's disease and other related conditions. To help you remember better, try some of these memory strategies.

1.   **Pay attention.** Instead of doing things habitually or on autopilot, pay close attention to what you are doing. If you deliberately avoid distractions, it is easier to pay attention. For example, when you shampoo your hair, make sure you pay attention to whether you use the conditioner, or you may forget if you used it or not. "Mindfulness" is a concept that helps us become aware of the present moment and can help us slow down our thoughts.

2.   **Form habits for things that are frequently misplaced or lost.** Rehearse and repeat. For example, use the same pocket or hook to store your keys when they are not in use. Make a deliberate attempt to remember a new phone number through repetition. Divide a longer number into chunks. Keep your medications or supplements organized and in a place that will help you remember to take them.

3. **Learn the strategy of association or cues.** To help memorize something new, such as a person's name, think of something that reminds you of him or her. For example, think of someone else you know (or knew) who has that name and match an associated feature with the new person. For example, my new neighbour's name is Maria. I also know a coworker named Maria. They are both short in stature. So, now, when I see Maria outside, I will remember her name.

4. **Know your learning style.** Get a good start on retaining new information by knowing what your preferred style of learning is. For some people, it helps to write things down. For others, they need to hear it. Some need to feel it. Some need to move it or actually do it. Maybe it's a combination of the above. For some, that may include an aid such as a notebook (paper or electronic), alarm clock, or calendar.

5. **Remain physically active.** Keeping the blood pumping throughout our bodies helps bring oxygen to our brain. Healthy brains need oxygen to thrive. To help keep your memory skills sharp, keep the blood flowing. Even taking a daily short, brisk walk is helpful!

There are some excellent books and other resources on protecting our brains and reducing our risk of developing dementia. Here are two books I have found helpful: *Outsmarting Alzheimer's: What You Can Do to Reduce Your Risk*, by Kenneth S. Kosik, M.D. (2015) and *The Memory Cure: How to Protect Your Brain Against Memory Loss and Alzheimer's Disease*, by Majid Fotuhi, M.D., Ph. D. (2003).

Although there are many other things we can do to improve and enhance our memory skills and brain health (such as learn a new musical instrument or language), the above five tips can help you get started. If you or someone you know is concerned about brain health or dementia, contact a healthcare professional for further assessment and possible treatment options.

If you are going to do only one thing for your brain health, make sure it is physical exercise. I went through this subject in more detail in the Physical Wellness chapter. What is good for your heart is good for your brain.

It is natural for our thinking skills to slow down as we age. We may have the occasional glitch in our memory. It is not natural or normal for us to lose the ability to think, process, remember, and utilize information in a functional way. It's not normal to start having a change in our personality. It's not normal to start "seeing things" or becoming paranoid. If you feel you are having more difficulties than what is to be expected, please make an appointment to talk to your doctor, and ask for an assessment of your cognitive functioning and overall mental health. You may even fit into the "Worried Well" category. There is nothing wrong with being proactive. Word-finding difficulties are concerning for some. Many other factors can affect your brain functioning, such as depression, delirium, vitamin deficiencies, medication side effects, alcohol or substance use, medical conditions, sleep disorders, stress, and many others.

If you are feeling good mentally and cognitively, keep up what you are doing. If not, I invite you to consider making some changes to improve your overall brain health.

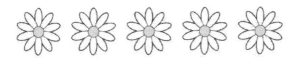

Brain-Wellness Self-Assessment

On a scale of 1 to 4, 1 being very dissatisfied, 4 being very satisfied, where are you at in terms of satisfaction with your cognition?

Circle one:

1 = Very dissatisfied. Horrible. Nonexistent.
2 = Dissatisfied. Not that great.
3 = Satisfied. It's okay.
4 = Very satisfied. Very content. Happy.

Brain-Wellness Reflection

If you score on the bottom half of the scale, what can you do, moving forward, to improve your cognition score? And when do you want to start making changes? How important is this to you? If you are scoring in the top half of the scale, what can you do to move toward a "four"?

Affirmations

- I have a good attitude towards growing older.
- I wear a helmet to protect my head as appropriate for a given activity.
- I play games and learn new things that stimulate my brain.
- I will seek help from a mental-health professional if I need it.
- I am eating healthily to nourish my brain.
- If my personality changes and people are saying I am difficult to get along with, I will see my doctor.
- I am open to learning new things.

Things to Try

- Sign up for a course to learn about something you are interested in.
- Do some memory tests to see where you are.
- If you feel like you are having trouble with your memory, make an appointment with your doctor.
- Commit to regular exercise to keep the oxygen pumping to your brain.
- Download an app that is good for the brain (e.g., learn a new language).
- Read up on foods that are good for healthy brain
- functioning.

References

Heart and Stroke. "Lifestyle risk factors." <u>Heartandstroke.ca/heart-disease-risk-and-prevention</u>. Retrieved 14 Jan 2021

Chapter 6

Social Wellness

*Deep human connection is...the purpose and result of a
meaningful life—and it will inspire the most amazing
acts of love, generosity, and humanity.*

— Melinda Gates

One of the basic needs of humans (other than food, clothing, and shelter) is the need to feel loved and like we belong—*belonging* in the sense that we feel connected and accepted by others. Social wellness is driven by the need for belonging and social connection, which evolves across the lifespan. The National Wellness Institute defines wellness as an active process through which people become aware of, and make choices towards, a more successful existence. When it comes to social wellness, the ability to form and maintain positive relationships, we all have a different level of need—some need more, and some need less.

I have seen many people who feel lonely, and I believe it has to do with the fact that they don't feel like they belong. This drive for wanting to belong never goes away and is present at all stages of our lifespan. It could be as simple as desiring a connection with one other person, such as a family member, friend, or a service provider in social services or healthcare. Simply joining a once-weekly "Adult Day Program" can significantly improve a person's overall wellness. These social programs offer much in terms of personal connections, social outings, and a regular dose of interpersonal activities. Having an excursion to look forward to can greatly enhance a once-lonely person's life. It doesn't really take much.

Fostering a sense of belonging goes both ways. For example, if we go to a family gathering or a social outing, we may or may not feel like we belong, based on our actions or the actions of others. For example, do you feel connected to others there? Who do you belong to? Do you feel accepted? Do you willingly and freely accept those in the group, or do you tend to disconnect? Do you accept others as they are, or do you judge or avoid them?

Sometimes our motivation for socialization is lacking due to mental-health problems such as depression or dementia. Others say they "like their own company" and were never "joiners." Social anxiety or lack of confidence can hinder initiating visits. Perhaps the person has a phobia or fear of being out in public (agoraphobia). Sometimes a loss can trigger our sense of connectedness in this world. We can improve our need for belonging by becoming self-aware and taking a good look at our life. We may need to be prepared to make some changes or even seek some professional help.

If we are fortunate enough to be born into and raised in a family that helps us feel loved and cared for, that is one thing. However, if we are born into a family that lacks the love and protection we need, we may feel abandoned, anxious, or rejected, and have trouble managing healthy relationships.

Those of us who were emotionally abandoned or abused in our younger years may not have developed a sense of what "love" is. We may crave and search for that feeling of acceptance and being cherished. We may search for this in relationships presented to us, such as in teachers, other relatives, and peers. Perhaps a series of romantic relationships helps fill the need for being loved. Sometimes these relationships are good and helpful. Other times they are abusive, empty, and unfulfilling. Our needs can be met positively through these other relationships as long as they are healthy and free from abuse.

Unhealthy Relationships

Sometimes we find comfort, acceptance, and connection through unhealthy relationships. Until we are mature enough to figure out what is emotionally and spiritually healthy for us, we may end up learning the hard way. Insults to our self-esteem can wear us down, which can lead to other unhealthy relationships. That is why it is so important for families (no matter what the family consists of, such as a single parent) to pay attention to their children's basic emotional and spiritual needs.

As we mature, we learn what is healthy and unhealthy. As teenagers, we may end up in troubling relationships to gain the love and acceptance we are innately or instinctually craving. We may end up getting involved with the "wrong crowd" because we feel understood and accepted.

The Problems With Social Isolation and Loneliness

We also know that loneliness and isolation are linked to depression. Depression is linked to dementia. Sometimes it's not clear what came first, the depression or the lack of connection to others. Sometimes depression is triggered by a loss or other traumatic event. Some people need to see a healthcare practitioner or mental-health specialist to determine if medication and psychotherapy can help.

Do You Feel Like You Belong? (Self-Assessment)

In some ways, we are all pieces of a puzzle, and most of us want to "fit in." If you answer "Yes" to any of the following questions (modified from the Sense of Belonging Instrument SOBI-P), then you may want to explore some ways to seek connection, so you feel a better sense of belonging:

1. It often feels like there is no place here on Earth where I truly fit in.

2. I don't fit in with my friends.

3. I feel like a misfit in most social situations.

4. I don't feel accepted by most people.

5. I could disappear for days, and my family or friends wouldn't miss me.

6. I tend to observe life rather than participate in it.

7. I feel left out of things.

Our need for intimacy, love, and romantic escapades starts when we are in the throes of teenagehood. We usually go through casual dating and a couple of serious relationships to know what we like or don't like when it comes to a life partner. Most of us will marry or cohabitate with our significant other and have children. Perhaps we will have someone to grow old with—enjoy a long-term marriage (50-plus years)—and live "happily ever after." Some may choose to be polyamorous, having more than one intimate relationship where all parties are in agreement.

It seems to me that married older men are happier than their wives. It also appears that women living alone seem to be happier than men who are on their own. Half of all of us who marry will end up separated or divorced. Not the greatest statistics. And all of us will end up alone in our life, due to the natural course of life. Widowed women end up alone longer than their male counterparts. Some of us will be on marriage or common-law relationship number two, or three, or more. Others will choose to remain alone, deciding that marriage or living with someone is not for us. No matter what we choose, the truth remains. We are social beings who thrive on sharing and caring. We laugh and cry together. Joy shared increases tenfold. Sorrow is lessened when shared with others.

Friendships

True friends are priceless. We need friends we can trust and share our lives with. Acquaintances come and go, but real friends are usually there for the long haul. An acquaintance may be a neighbour or a cashier at your local grocery store. Childhood friends are those with whom we share history. It's usually easier to trust someone you have known for a long time. Best friends are those we share a lot in common with and the people we can confide in.

There are all kinds of friends—even ones who aren't the greatest. You know, the ones who "dump" on us? The person who tells you all the bad stuff that's going on in her life? I call those friends "Dumpers." Then there is the Once-a-Year friend (someone you may see yearly for their birthday or a special occasion), the Friend with Kids, the Mentor, the Work friend, and the Sports friend. Friends who are lots of fun are the Partying, Shopping, Dining, and Crazy-Shit friends (the person who is willing to do crazy, fun things like zip lining!). There are the friends you like to travel with, and the friends you went to school with. You may have a friend or two who will call you on things and challenge you—ultimately helping you grow (spouses are good at that, too!). If we are lucky to have friends like these, we are blessed. Friends help us feel like we belong.

Similar to a person who is stuck in an abusive relationship, you may have friends who drag you down. Sometimes it's easier to avoid conflict or deal with your problems, so these bad relationships continue. You may be afraid of hurting someone's feelings, or perhaps you have had this friend for a long time, so you just "put up with it." Some women feel it's better to have a "bad friend" than no friend at all.

If you have so-called friends that bring you down and empty your bucket rather than fill it, it may be time to think about the relationship and what it means to you. How do you feel after you have been with that person? Do you feel full of energy, or do you feel depleted? Do you feel fulfilled, or do you feel agitated? Happy or unhappy? Notice patterns with certain people. If you notice a negative feeling almost every time you have interaction with that person, then maybe it's time to cut your ties or at least take a break. I call this "Cleaning out your closet." If you have an issue with someone, and you have asked them to treat you better, it's best to disengage. Ultimately, we teach people how to treat us, and it's up to us who we want in our circle. Unhealthy relationships can affect our social well-being. This can spill over into other areas of our lives. Moving on from unhealthy relationships makes room for new ones.

The same goes for unhealthy family relationships. Whether it's a blood relative, or a relative through marriage (in-laws), good relationships are not guaranteed. Many family conflicts can cause irreparable rifts. I know of many situations where the family members don't talk to each other. There are also situations in which family members become strangers—and estrangement occurs. I have spoken to one too many older adults who are estranged from their son or daughter. It is heartbreaking when parents don't know what they did to cause the distancing. Seeking resolution at the end of life is near impossible, especially when no contact has been made for many years. The desire to mend these estranged relationships becomes more intense for some people as they get older. Perhaps it is the need to repair the broken or non-existing ties to feel complete. Like they belong.

If you feel there is a need for reconciliation, problem-solving, or mediation, consider pursuing family or couples therapy with a qualified professional.

Pets

Pets can enrich our lives in more ways than we realize. Our pets can provide us with unconditional love, companionship, something to "look after," and emotional support when we are feeling down. Dogs are a big responsibility, but having a buddy or a cuddle when we feel lonesome or sad offers a great way to cope.

I have never had a cat, but my son and his significant other have two. They adopted them when they were kittens. They say the cats provide them with endless laughs and entertainment. I have had all kinds of pets in my lifetime, including turtles, birds, guinea pigs, hamsters, fish (if you can call them pets!). Dogs have always been a big part of my life. The first dog I had was a black lab named Tina. She was so sweet and gentle. She was a perfect family dog, and she was big enough that I could use her as a pillow.

Dogs can also get us outside and walking. Off-leash dog parks are fun places where your dog can run free, and you can meet up with other people for a chat (you have something in common!). There are dog play-groups and doggy daycares that your dogs can enjoy. And don't forget obedience classes. That's always a good idea, especially if you have never been a dog owner before. Therapy dogs can help people feel good. I've seen them at airports and in long-term care homes. I saw one at the university and the hospital, too. Watchdogs can help protect your home or alert you when someone is on your property. Some people let their dogs sleep on their beds. There are mixed reviews on this, so I say, if you want your dog on your bed, be prepared to give up some space!

Lifelong Need for Belonging

The need to feel like we belong never goes away, just like our need for water and safety. We are social beings. We depend on others. We do things in groups. Our connections to others change as we grow and become wiser. Our individual personality traits remain the same, but our values and morals may change over time. Having children and starting our own families usually wakes up our moral compass. What is right and wrong suddenly become clear.

Our own innate need for belonging is often met by having children. Young children usually offer unconditional love and acceptance (Spoiler alert: Things will change as they become more independent!). Our small and sometimes growing family helps us meet our needs for feeling loved and like we belong.

Friends can help provide a sense of belonging for those who don't have children, pets, or other relatives (such as nieces/nephews).

Intergenerational relationships are invaluable. Our children may eventually have children of their own. Being a grandparent is a wonderful experience (from what I've heard!). Caring for one's grandchildren can be very rewarding (and exhausting!). The connection between a grandchild and a grandparent is a special one.

My grandparents were special to me, and they helped me learn what it's like to get older. I taught them new things I was learning in school. We can encourage relationships between different generations, ultimately helping one generation be more understanding and connected to the other. For example, a nursing home may have a daycare provider come to visit. Or there may be a housing project that has young adults looking after and for older adults. They can learn from and support one another. Ultimately, this leads to less ageism and more acceptance towards each other.

As we age, it is likely we will find ourselves in a caregiving situation. Our aging or ailing relatives or parents will most likely need some kind of support at some point. Most people like to think they will remain independent up until their dying day. I have seen how the years can affect a person's ability to manage independently, despite their efforts to resist help. Dependence on others—and the ability and willingness of others to provide help—is at the root of caregiving; it is an intimate social connection.

Most people are independent and self-sufficient once they reach a certain level of maturity. For my children, that meant around age 16. Up until then, they required an increased level of care and nurturing. At times, the demands of caring for them was trying, and I felt the stress of being a working mother. Luckily for me, I had an equal partner in caring for these children (my husband). The need for a caregiver eventually fades. The role of the parent or guardian changes, and although there is a social and interpersonal connection, the responsibilities are different.

After the children move out, there is a transition period. A sense of loss may be felt, and then an adjustment to the empty nest is made. Sometimes they come back—"Boomerang" kids. Grandchildren offer newness, hope, and excitement. I have heard so many good things about being a grandparent. It appears to be a wonderful time, especially when the children are very young.

At some point, in our later years, there becomes a need for another pair of helping hands (or two). At times, it becomes difficult to navigate through the complexities of life. Physical or cognitive impairments can make it challenging to deal with certain tasks. Going to the doctor's office for a checkup can become overwhelming if we are no longer able to drive. Merely getting to the doctor's office can become a challenge. Where exactly is the specialist's office? How long is the walk from the parking lot going to be? All of these concerns and others can be enough to make us stay at home.

Caregiving

Caregivers—those who provide care and support—are invaluable members of society. They offer physical and emotional support to those who need a little (or a lot of) help. They can be instrumental in providing practical support and advice. Caregivers can be formal (such as nurses or healthcare aids) or informal (such as family members, friends, neighbours, or volunteers). The task of caregiving can be both physically and emotionally exhausting, however, it can also be gratifying.

In my clinical work, I always take the time to determine who the primary, or most important, supporters are in my older clients' lives. I always ask, "Who is the person you would call if you needed help?" or "Who can you count on if you ran into trouble?" I determine whom they frequently speak to or spend the most time with. These are the primary caregivers. I also try to figure out who the back-up or secondary caregivers are, too—just in case.

It is important to note who the caregivers are and to acknowledge the help and support they provide to the "caree" (the person they give care to). I also find it important to ask how the caregivers are doing and if they have stress in their lives. Is looking after spouse, mom, dad, sibling, or others causing them any stress? If so, is there some kind of help or other suggestion I could offer to help lessen the load? For example, if it is becoming too much to clean Mom's apartment, could they try hiring someone to do that for her? Or, if it is becoming too much of a battle to get a loved one into the shower, could someone else take over this task?

Caregivers, those who give care, also need to be permitted to care for themselves. They should be encouraged to take "mini-vacations" or extended vacations. However, they don't need to be pressured into this, as that can also cause added strain on their already-busy schedules. The main idea is to help prevent burnout. If caregivers don't look after themselves, then who will? And if they become burnt out or sick, who will look after their loved one? At that point, there will be a need for more caregivers to look after them as well.

In my helping professional role, I had developed a relationship with Margaret. She was caring for her husband, Bill, who had dementia. Margaret had every opportunity to tell me she felt overwhelmed, but she insisted she was doing fine. One day I called Margaret, and there was no answer. I had trouble reaching her, so I called her daughter, Cathy. She informed me that her mom had had a stroke and was in the hospital. Cathy had to look after her dad while her mom was getting tests done. Cathy said her mom thinks she "stroked out" because she was so stressed looking after her husband all on her own. The stroke could have happened whether she was receiving help or not, but she recognized it was very stressful for her, and it most likely was a factor in triggering her health crisis. Fortunately, Cathy's mom recovered and was able to return home. With the help of Home Care, Cathy and Margaret put together a plan that included more support for Bill.

Encouraging caregivers to care for themselves is just as important as ensuring the older person's needs are met. Taking time, even if it is a "stolen moment," to take a deep breath, read a chapter of that new book, or walk around the block is crucial to the caregiver's overall well-being. If caregivers know they are not alone, they will feel supported, and that will help give them the strength and motivation to continue doing what they are doing. Feeling they belong to a community of caregivers will help them see the rewards and benefits of their efforts. It may also inspire them to care for themselves.

I find that those who feel a sense of belonging have good connections with others through family, friendships, and other social relationships. They also know who to avoid, based on the way they are treated. Friendships and family relationships can be—and need to be—fostered and nurtured.

There are other ways to give back to our communities. Donations to charities, volunteering, organizing fundraising events, or participating in other worthy causes can help us feel connected. We are social beings, and a good balance of give and take can foster a healthy sense of social connectedness and well-being. Need a boost? Help someone else out, or do them a favour. Giving of ourselves and of our time to help others can increase our happiness and well-being.

What I have learned over the years of working with older adults and their caregivers is that family members are often the main source of love, meaning, and belonging. If this is not possible, or if people feel they want more, the workplace and social- or religious-based clubs and other groups can help fulfill these needs. If there isn't a group, make one! I know of a man who lived in an assisted-living residence with a pool table. He needed some buddies to play with, so he organized a tournament!

Examples of groups and other social opportunities (virtual, by phone, and in-person for olders include:

- Senior Centres
- Exercise Classes
- Educational Events
- Retirement Communities
- Interest Groups (e.g., knitting, quilting, gardening, astronomy, genealogy, photography)
- Church/Synagogue or other Spiritual Based Groups
- Cultural Clubs
- Women's Groups (e.g., Red Hat Ladies, Crown Jewels of Canada Society, Circle of Friends)
- Men's Sheds (a movement that started in Australia in 2007; sheds are for groups of men to do things together such as woodworking, bike repairs, and cooking)

Most programs for older adults are very accommodating and aware of challenges that may be encountered. Just remember that, if limitations exist, there are workarounds. For example, people who have a hearing impairment can wear hearing aids or sit close to whoever is speaking. If someone can't afford transportation to get to the program, ask if there is some kind of financial support or volunteer program. If you use a walker or need a wheelchair and the place isn't accessible, bring it to the organizers' attention and suggest an alternative.

Having an internet connection and knowing how to use a computer, tablet, or smartphone can also help keep people connected. Email and texting are easy to learn. Facebook or other social-media sites can help keep family and friends connected. You can meet lots of new people as well. I have hundreds of friends worldwide due to our mutual interests and the incredible magic of the world wide web. I have connected with others through LinkedIn (a social-media site for professionals and those seeking work and professional collaboration), Facebook, and Instagram. Other popular sites such as Pinterest, Reddit, and Twitter are places one can go to find like-minded individuals. We never know what new and exciting platform is around the corner, so we may just want to remain open to the possibilities. (I hesitated to put down the sites I use and know of, as I know these trends change so fast. Vine came and went; now TikTok is popular. We just have to be ready for change at all times!)

To end isolation and loneliness brought on by a sense of "not belonging" or feeling left out takes some effort, and it goes both ways. Sometimes it takes a little boost of confidence and "guts" to get yourself out there. To improve your sense of belonging, you need to help others feel like *they* belong, to allow that connection and acceptance to grow.

Our basic human need and motivation for feeling like we belong in this world can be nurtured and supported by our actions. The reverse is also true. Think about *who* you belong to, *what* you belong to, and *who* and *what* belongs to you. If you want to increase your sense of connection and acceptance, it will take some effort. It's the same as securing food, water, clothing, shelter, and safety. It doesn't happen all on its own. I encourage you to take stock and ensure your relationships are healthy and fulfilling.

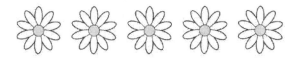

Social-Wellness Self-Assessment

On a scale of 1 to 4, 1 being very dissatisfied, 4 being very satisfied, where are you at in terms of satisfaction with your social wellness?

Circle one:

1 = Very dissatisfied. Horrible. Nonexistent.
2 = Dissatisfied. Not that great.
3 = Satisfied. It's okay.
4 = Very satisfied. Very content. Happy.

Social-Wellness Reflection

If you score on the bottom half of the scale, what can you do, moving forward, to improve your Social Wellness score? And when do you want to start making changes? How important is this to you? If you are scoring in the top half of the scale, what can you do to move toward a "four"?

Affirmations

- I am seeking and nurturing healthy connections with others.
- I belong to someone.
- Someone belongs to me.
- As a caregiver, I am also caring for myself.
- I have healthy relationships.
- I can get or give a hug whenever I want to.
- I acknowledge others' birthdays and other important dates.
- I belong to some great groups.
- I love my pets, and they are great to have around.
- I am satisfied with my friendships.
- I tell my friends how much they mean to me.
- I appreciate my life partner.
- I have friends I can count on.
- I like my social network.

Things to Try

- Take stock of all your relationships, and decide if it's time to "Clean out your closet."
- Call a friend or family member to ask *how* they are doing, and ask them tell you about *what* they are doing. Make sure you and the other person get equal time to talk. Share news and views about yourself, your own family, and your own life, however, ensure they talk about their life, too.
- Tell your partner how much you care.
- Send a greeting card to a friend.
- Join a social group for fun.
- Volunteer for a cause you are interested in.
- Visit a shelter or adopt a pet.
- Find a job you enjoy with a boss and co-workers you can relate to.
- Try out a club that is focused on one of your interests, and see if you feel like you belong.

- Contribute to newsletters and share your expertise with others.
- Plan an outing or a visit with someone you care about or would like to get to know better.
- Write a letter to someone.
- Join a social-media site like Facebook, and find some groups you are interested in.
- Join a support group.
- Seek a counsellor if you are stuck and want to make some positive changes in your life

---

References

Nolan, Laurence C. (2011). "Dimensions of Aging and Belonging for the Older Person and the Effects of Ageism." http://digitalcommons.law.byu.edu/cgi/viewcontent.cgi?article=1451&context=jpl.

National Wellness Institute: https://nationalwellness.org

Other Resources

For more information on caregivers, check out the "Portrait of Caregivers" (2012) from Statistics Canada.

For additional reading, see "Maslow's Hierarchy of Needs" (such as in: http://www.simplypsychology.org/maslow.html)

Chapter 7

Sexual Wellness

*Sex appeal is 50% what you've got
and 50% what people think you've got.*

— Sophia Loren

Sex, sexuality, sex appeal (attractiveness), and feminine power are topics that often get ignored when it comes to women and aging. We must not forget about our sexuality, as it is part of our core essence. I believe that sexuality should have its own category when it comes to the dimensions of wellness. Sex is and has been considered a taboo subject in North America. However, sexuality is an integral part of our being. We are born male or female, which is one of the main drivers of our behaviour and instincts. Some are born intersex, where there are facets of both the female and male organs inside and out. Our species' survival depends on the sexual act. We remain sexual beings all of our lives.

Sexuality is a word we use to talk about how we understand our bodies and how we understand our relationships. This understanding includes all aspects of who we are—our values and beliefs, bodies, desires, relationships, gender, and our thoughts and feelings about all of these. Because our sexuality is made up of so many different components, our understanding of our sexuality is ever-changing and unique to each person.

The most important thing to understand about sexuality is that it is self-defined, that is, that every person is allowed to talk about and understand their own sexuality in their own way that makes sense to them. Sexuality is dynamic and always changing; often, we may discover that different parts of our lives may interact with each other in confusing or affirming ways. This is okay and is part of our normal development. Exploring our own sexuality, rooted within the principles of consent and sexual rights, is a key determinant of our health and wellness.

— Sexuality Education Resource Centre Manitoba

The only times I have been asked about sex is the occasional discussion with a doctor or a friend. As a geriatric clinician (working with and for adults aged 65 and older), I don't even ask about sexuality and intimacy during the assessment. It's completely missing from the list of questions we ask! Paradoxically, we live in a culture that exploits sexuality and jokes about it frequently. For some, it is an embarrassing or shameful subject. It is pervasive, and not only does "sex sell," but pornography is rampant on the internet.

"Sex-Positive" Approach to Aging

Sex positivity is an important ideology that acknowledges and affirms each person's right to experience and define their sexuality throughout their lifetime in whatever way they choose. Grounded in comprehensive sexuality and sexual-health education, sex positivity is inclusive and respectful of a wide range of sexual experiences, expressions, consensual activities (including non-activity), and identities (including asexuality). A sex-positive approach realizes the potentially life-enhancing aspects of human sexuality and presents sexuality as something that can be valued and celebrated, thereby giving people permission to consider their own sexuality.

It is important to note that sex positivity is not sex promotion. The movement does not dictate that everyone

98

must enjoy or be interested in sex. Further, sex-positivity does not place moral judgments on whether people are interested in or enjoy sex. Rather, sex positivity allows space for people to consider their sexuality, and encourages discussion about a wide range of sexuality-related topics.

— Sexuality Education Resource Centre Manitoba

Sex-negativity approaches sex and sexuality from a place of fear. Sex-positivity encourages the promotion of an open and progressive attitude towards sex and sexuality. Sexually transmitted infections (STIs) should be destigmatized in order to promote a safer environment for people to have sex, get tested without shame, and to freely share their status with their partners. A sex-positive society accepts polyamory

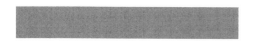

Shower with a sex partner!

(more than one relationship that is known to all), kinks (unusual sexual preferences), and hookup culture (a casual sexual encounter).

Sexual orientation is the term used for the gender a person is attracted to. A woman may be attracted to men, other women, or both, therefore, she may be heterosexual, homosexual, or bisexual, respectively. The same goes for men. A newer term, "pansexual," describes people who don't have any limitations in their sexual orientation when it comes to male or female. Homosexuality used to be less accepted than it is now, and many people are "coming out" and stating their sexual preferences. Same-sex relationships are more prevalent on television, in movies, and in the general public. The "Gay Pride" movement helps to support people who identify as Lesbian, Gay, Bisexual, Transgender, or Queer (LGBTQ) and end the violence and discrimination experienced by them. Older people who are homosexual are still struggling with "coming out" due to previous stigma and perhaps the way they were treated.

Unless you are asexual, that is, without any sexual feelings or associations, sex is an integral part of life. It is nothing to be ashamed of or embarrassed about. The more we talk about it, the more we can support each other.

> The Sexuality Education Resource Centre defines sex as an activity in which one, two, or more people use words or touch to arouse themselves and or each other.

> Every person can define what a sexual act means for them. Sex might involve touching genitals, but it might not. Sex for somebody might mean cuddling with clothes on or sending a sexy text message. It is essential that every person involved in the sexual activity gets consent from the other people involved before any sexual touching or sexual talking happens.

> There are many reasons two or more people might want to engage in sexual activity with each other. SERC likes to talk about pleasure being at the centre of sexual activity. Though there are many reasons people may want to engage in sexual activity with each other, it is important that everybody involved feels good in the interaction and that consent is present. We like to highlight the idea that sex, sexual touching, and sexy talking should feel good and safe for everybody involved.

> — Sexuality Education Resource Centre Manitoba

People can be, and are, sexually active into late adulthood. I often refer to information on the Mayo Clinic website (www.mayoclinic.org), and they have some great articles on "Senior Sex: Tips for Older Men" and "Sexual Health and Aging: Keep the Passion Alive." At the time of printing this book, there was no section called "Tips for Older Women." Check those articles out if you have a chance. They describe the issues that may come up, and they also give some great advice.

One good thing about being older and having sex is that you don't have to worry about getting pregnant. If you are a woman who has not had her period for 12 months (menopause), then there is no need for birth control. However, if you are having sexual intercourse, it's imperative that for vaginal-penile sex, a condom is used to help prevent the risk of contracting a sexually transmitted infection (STI). The unfortunate news is that STIs are on the rise among older adults, specifically syphilis, chlamydia, and gonorrhea. Additionally, the human papillomavirus (HPV) is a common sexually transmitted infection that can lead to cancer of the cervix, throat, anus, and other related areas. The HPV vaccine is available to help prevent infection and is most effective when given to youth (before sexual activity) or people in their earlier adult years.

We don't ask when people age out of
singing or eating ice cream;
why would we stop making love?

— Ashton Applewhite, *This Chair Rocks: A Manifesto Against Ageism*

One of the interesting things I have learned about our current generation is that people are "grooming" their pubic hairs. It is no longer cool to have an unruly bush like it was back in the old days. Look up "How to Trim Pubic Hair" on the internet, and you will get all kinds of ideas. The Brazilian Wax looks pretty intense, where all (or almost all) the pubic hair is removed. Men are doing it, too. "Manscaping" is a term used by men who trim or remove the hair on their bodies.

Some women may experience sexual freedom in their middle years. They may start to feel more lively and spirited. Their libido may have increased. Women who are mothers of older children find more time to focus on themselves and what gives them pleasure. I have heard the term "sassy" to describe middle-aged women. One of my good friends talked about getting her "Mojo" back. Some women feel more confident as they age and become sexually curious. They may start to watch soft porn or read erotica. They may experiment with sex toys, including vibrators.

Keep in mind, as we get older, we may require more sexual stimulation for desired effect. Sex is all about having fun and relaxing. If the goal is to have an orgasm, then the pressure may be too great, and it may not be achieved.

Sexy-Time Ideas for You

♦ Host a sex-toy party, or visit a sex shop.
♦ Choose a good sex partner with whom you can experiment.
♦ Try "sexting" your lover.
♦ Write a sexy story.
♦ Ensure you are communicating your needs with your partner, as he or she is likely unable to read your mind.
♦ Be adventurous with your partner, and try using ice cubes or feathers on erogenous zones.
♦ Consider getting a remote-controlled sex toy that can be turned on and off by your lover, who is somewhere else in the house.
♦ Make out in a different area of the house or in a vehicle.
♦ Engaging in slow dancing or massage can get the love hormones flowing.

Expressing our needs, desires, and wants to our sex partners can enhance our experience and the connection. As Joan Price who wrote *Naked at Our Age* states, "Talking about sex with a partner (whether committed, casual, or anything in between) is not something our generation learned (or practiced). But it's never too late to learn to do it, and it does enhance relationships. Writing down what you want to say helps if the words disappear or get caught in your throat when you try to speak them."

Menopausal Effects

Menopause is something that all women go through. It is a time when they no longer menstruate or have periods. It is the end of the childbearing years. I have read that a woman is not officially through the menopause transition or post-menopausal until she has not had a period for one year. The time before menopause, or perimenopause, can last for a few months to a few years. The average age of menopause is fifty-one. Some women have difficulties going through this transition. Some of the most common experiences include sleep problems, weight gain, thinning hair, dry skin, loss of breast fullness, hot flashes, chills, night sweats, vaginal dryness, and emotional changes. I know this to be a fact because I went through menopause at age 50, and I experienced most of these symptoms. Women can seek help from a doctor or a gynecologist if these symptoms cause too much grief or disrupt their lives (such as not being able to sleep). There are many books written on the subject, and I like Dr. Christine Northrup's approach. Check out her books for more information, or find another professional who can recommend you some current, reliable resources.

Attractiveness

When it comes to attractiveness, we can consider not only our outward appearance but how we feel inside. Some people exude confidence, which can be attractive to others. Those who are too confident can come across as "cocky" or arrogant. There is a delicate balance between being overly confident and just the right amount of being sure of yourself.

Women are often judged by how they look. I am a former (small-town) beauty-pageant winner. At a young age, I learned how to look and act so people would admire my feminine beauty. My mother was a former child model, so she taught me how to hold in my stomach, put on makeup, and make sure my hair looked nice. She was always giving me beauty advice. We had many fights about potato chips, as she was okay with my younger brothers eating them but discouraged me from having them. She didn't want me to get fat—as slim was more beautiful at the time. I learned a lot from her about body image and valuing attractiveness, which she learned from her mother. I am passing on the same values to my daughter, although we don't fight about potato chips (other than her finding my secret stash!).

I entered my first beauty pageant when I was sixteen. I won the "Miss Draft Horse" title and then competed in the "Emo Fair" in Northwestern Ontario. I finished as runner-up in the Emo Fair pageant. Then, at nineteen, I was encouraged to compete in the "Miss Fort Frances" pageant—and I won. I went on to be one of the contestants in the "Miss Canada Pageant" in Toronto in October 1985. I didn't win or even come close, but it was quite the experience. I learned all about modeling, women competing against each other, and "catty" behaviour. The girl who won the year I was in the Miss Canada Pageant was Rene Newhouse, and she was lovely. I have two scrapbooks on my pageant days, and I have kept a letter from Rene. I am glad she won.

My pageant experiences helped me develop confidence. In the eighties, women were very much judged on their physical appearance. Pageant competitions have changed their focus somewhat. Some are even cancelled!

I encourage confidence-building in my daughter in different ways. For example, she did very well in school, and she was an athlete and played for an elite volleyball team. I foster confidence in a healthy and balanced way for her (as well as my son). By the way, my daughter was never interested in beauty pageants whatsoever.

When I was in my early 30s, I learned a lot about bras. I worked part-time at The Bra Bar and Panterie in Winnipeg. We sold bras, panties, and other lingerie. I am a trained "Bra-fitter extraordinaire." Many women are not aware of how a bra should fit. They may have the wrong cup or band size. There is no standardization for bra manufacturing, so there are many companies, and you may find one brand fits you better than the others. I have my favourite brands for both underwire and wireless.

Wearing the correct size and fit of bra can make "your girls" look good—immediately improving how your clothes fit. I believe it's worth going to a nice shop for a proper bra-fitting experience. Bras come in all colours, prints, and price ranges, and sometimes there are nice panties to match! Wearing a pretty matching bra and panty set can make you feel sexy. I find the older I get, the more I go for comfort. In my opinion, a nice padded, wireless bra is very comfy.

While we are on the topic of physical attractiveness (sex appeal), there are a couple of things I have noticed in older people. For men, I notice that hair starts to change locations. For example, they may start to have a receding hairline or begin to go bald while the hair in their noses and ears start growing. Even eyebrows start to look unruly. If I had to give some advice to men as they age, I would advise them to make sure they keep their facial hair trimmed and neat and remove any unwanted unruly hair from the nose and ears. I find it very distracting talking to a man who has hairs growing where they normally don't.

I was 47 when I noticed my near-vision skills were starting to become a problem. I found myself needing "reading" glasses, so I found some cheap ones at the local dollar store. These helped tremendously. I wear makeup, so I started to notice I was having difficulty putting on my eye makeup. Putting on eyeliner and mascara takes a certain amount of skill and near-vision! I noticed how much I loved a lighted magnifying makeup mirror at a hotel I stayed at. It made it so much easier to put on my eye makeup. I bought a stand-up mirror, which has made a big difference in how I put on my makeup now. I notice some middle-aged and older women with clumped mascara or eyeliner that appears too thick, and I wonder if they have ever tried a lighted magnifying mirror. I guess most likely not. If you love to wear makeup, I would strongly suggest you try one of these magical mirrors. Some people say they don't like them because they show all the imperfections in a big way. I say it's great because makeup can help hide those imperfections.

I also noticed I was starting to get those little hairs growing out of my nose, so I bought one of those nose hair trimmers a few years ago. It's a little battery-operated device. I also would suggest a great pair of tweezers to get rid of those tiny, annoying chin hairs.

Some women find that their eyebrows start to get very thin. Or, as in my case, they begin to go grey and get very light in colour. You can use an eyebrow pencil to fill them in or have them tattooed on. There are permanent and semi-permanent ways to have this done, with microblading or micropigmentation (make sure you are seen by a licensed professional if you decide to go this way).

For those concerned about thinning eyelashes, you can try using fake eyelashes or get semi-permanent eyelash extensions. This is generally an expensive and lengthy procedure, but it can be done regularly or occasionally for a special event. As an aside, those of us who use Lumigan medicated eye drops to treat glaucoma may find an interesting side effect of having longer and thicker eyelashes. I have noticed this in my practice with older adults. Those who use this medicated eye drop often have thicker and longer lashes than most people their age. I was once talking with an 85-year-old man who had the most beautiful eyelashes, top and bottom. I asked him if he uses Lumigan, and he said he did.

As we age, we develop lines and wrinkles on our faces and other parts of our bodies. This may be a big problem for women because we live in a society where youth is more valued. A simple moisturizing cream can help our skin feel soft and hydrated.

Celebrities and those who are usually in the public eye often have "work done." This beauty ideal is not achievable or desired by everyone due to the costs involved, and some people don't like the idea of altering their appearance. This is a personal decision that all people have a right to make. I stay away from judging people based on the fact that they have had "work done" or not.

Technically, people who colour their hair have had "work done," and I would never condemn anyone for that, either. The bottom line is people will do what they can or want to help them feel more at ease and confident with their appearance and body image. In the end, it's a personal choice.

There are ways to digitally alter and enhance how we look through using programs like "Photoshop." It is so easy nowadays with all the different computer programs and applications. Some filters can "soften" our look (reduce the look of wrinkles or other imperfections), and there are ways to minimize or enhance certain features. If you want to have a smaller waist or bigger breasts, it can be done easily with a computer. Digitally enhanced photos are often seen on magazine covers and sometimes even videos. Some celebrities are taking a stand and are speaking out against these altered images.

When I had my professional portrait taken at age 48 in 2014, the photographer said he would "soften" my photograph. I said I didn't want it softened, as I wanted my lines and imperfections to remain. I want to appear "real" and embrace my age. I want to be a role model for others and to say it's okay to grow older. On the flip side, it's okay to do any enhancements you might choose. We need to be more accepting of each other's journey through this life and not have the pressure to conform either way.

I have learned that it is common for people to lie about certain things on online dating sites. Some people lie about not only their height and weight but also about their age. It somehow makes us more attractive if we are younger. I don't think we have people making themselves out to be older than they are. The only time I did that was when I wanted to get into a bar when I was underage. I always share my actual age now, as I don't see any benefit in lying about it.

Double Standards

There are some double standards when it comes to aging and dating. There is the "Cougar." A cougar is a woman aged 35 and older who likes to pursue and attract younger men. What do you call a younger man who likes to date older women? Well, the best term I have heard of is "cougar hunter" or "cougar hawk." Then we have the "Gold Digger." This is a term usually referring to a younger woman who likes to date rich older men, i.e., "Sugar Daddies." The term "Gold Digger" is also applied to men who like to pursue "Sugar Mammas." What about the older man who leaves his wife for a younger lover who is as young as his own daughter? What about May-December romances? Isn't it okay to have differences? Must there always be an ulterior motive?

The most important sexual
organ is the brain.

— Natalie Wilton, Social Worker/Sex Therapist

Metabolism Changes

Changing metabolisms can alter our weight and body shape. The mid-life muffin top—that roll just above the waistline—is very common in older people. Maybe you've heard of "Love Handles?" "Beer belly" is a common term used for men who carry extra weight around their middle. There is a danger in carrying around an excess of "visceral" fat, as mentioned in the Physical Wellness chapter. Not only does it change our body image and self-perception, it also causes an increased health risk. Being in shape, maintaining a healthy body weight, and loving ourselves no matter what our body looks like are necessary attributes for a healthy and happy sex life.

Posture

Body posture is also part of looking and feeling great. Sitting up straight, walking tall, and looking forward can help improve our posture. As we age, our back can start to curve and cause us to walk with a stooped posture. This is called a kyphotic spine, and it is often the result of vertebral fractures (broken backbones) in the spine, causing an outward curve. Think the Hunchback of Notre Dame. Osteoporosis, or deterioration of the bones and tissue, can happen as we age due to hormonal changes or vitamin deficiencies. One can do exercises to help keep the bones and back strong, and a physiotherapist can help you with this. Seeking nutritional advice from a dietician can help ensure healthy and strong bones. Everyone is at risk for developing osteoporosis, however, older white women carry the highest risk. So, sit up straight, chin up, and take care of your back.

> **MEANING BEHIND THE LYRICS**
>
> The song that I connected with this Valentine's Day was 'Love Myself' by Hailee Steinfeld. *'I love me!/Gonna love myself/No, I don't need/anybody else!'* I love that song. Just today I was reading the lyrics and discovered it's about a woman pleasuring herself...OMG! Ha-ha! I'm all for self-pleasure. I initially thought it was about women's self-empowerment!
> — Teresa

Sexual Health

Sexual health and maintenance of our sexual organs and private parts is an essential part of our overall routine health checks. It is important for women to have a pap test (a screening for cervical cancer) every three years (perhaps more often, depending on your cancer risk). In the absence of having penile-vaginal intercourse, vaginal dilators, dildos, and "Battery Operated Boyfriends"—or BOB, as my gynecologist calls it—can help keep our vaginal canal healthy and can make the pap test procedure more tolerable. Vaginal stenosis or atrophy (shortening/narrowing) can make sex or pap tests uncomfortable. Vaginal lubricant is a must for many women. Some even choose to pursue pricy vaginal rejuvenation to correct age-related problems such as urinary incontinence or loosened vaginal tissue.

Breast-cancer screening can be done monthly as a self-examination of the breasts (checking for lumps), and a doctor can do a physical breast exam on a regular basis. Mammograms are recommended every two years for women aged 50 to 74 (again, it could be more often, depending on your cancer risk). Men are encouraged to check for breast cancer as well.

For men, one of the common problems I often hear about is an enlarged prostate. The prostate is a small gland in males which makes sperm. It often becomes enlarged in men as they age, and they have a condition called Benign Prostatic Hyperplasia (BPH). This does not make a man more at risk for prostate cancer. A man with BPH may find it harder to urinate or have trouble controlling his urine and becoming incontinent (can't control the flow of urine and have dribbling or full-out loss of control).

For men who have prostate cancer, treatments for this can affect their sexual functioning. It is a good idea for a man to discuss these risks in detail with a healthcare provider.

"Sex changes with aging, but for every problem, there is a solution," says Joan Price, "senior sexpert" for the older-than-fifty population.

Sexual Performance

The mechanical and physical requirements for penetrative vaginal sex require an erect penis and a healthy, welcoming vagina. Ill health, surgery, cancer treatment, hormonal changes, trauma, or medications are some of the reasons why penis-vagina sex isn't possible. Sometimes there are fixes for these problems. A pelvic-floor physiotherapist and gynecologist are good options for women when things aren't working "down there."

Men who have erectile dysfunction can have problems with getting and keeping an erection. Some medications can help with this.

Anxiety is a crippler. For men, it speeds up the sexual response cycle. For women, it slows it down.

The vaginal walls can become dry and thin for women, and there are lubricants that can help with that. Personal lubricants are used to help reduce friction and are also used for all types of sexual activity (including masturbation). There are different types of lubricants, and the main ones are based in water, silicone, or oil. There are also hybrid products that combine more than one type. It's a good idea to start with one type and then try another type if that one doesn't seem to work for you.

Women experiencing hormonal changes may also find a need for a vaginal lubricant. Consider hormone-free vaginal suppositories or ointments to help keep the vaginal area moist and healthy. Directions for the use of these products varies, so read the instructions carefully. Prescription creams and suppositories are options you can discuss with your doctor or gynecologist.

Self-Pleasure

Masturbation or self-stimulation is one form of expressing our sexuality in the same way dressing and being clean is. It is not a moral or religious issue. The Sexuality Education Resource Centre gives some information about the topic on their website (https://serc.mb.ca):

> Masturbation describes the action of touching and exploring your sexual body parts. Masturbation feels good to many people. It can also be a helpful way to learn about yourself, what kind of sexy touching you like, and what kind of sexy touching you don't like. It is important that you only masturbate in a private place for reasons of consent and respect to people around you.
>
> Every person is different; some people like to masturbate frequently, some people once in a while, and some people don't enjoy it at all. Some people like to masturbate only around their sexual partner(s). A person's desire to masturbate may change throughout their life. This is all

normal. There is no right amount of masturbating a person can do; it is completely up to them. The only time masturbation might be a concern is if it begins to affect a person's work, school, or personal life. In cases like these, you might consider seeing a counsellor or therapist, as masturbation should not negatively affect other parts of your life.

— Sexuality Education Resource Centre Manitoba

Fragrances

Another way to express yourself sexually and sensually is through fragrances. Although we see more and more people sensitive to fragrances in public places and workplaces, we are still seeing lots of fragrances being advertised and sold in stores and online. I was always a big fan of wearing perfume as a younger woman. I have been through many fragrances. I remember my mom wearing Chanel No. 5 and my grandmother wearing Youth-Dew from Estée Lauder. One of my favourites from years ago was called Beautiful, also from Estée Lauder.

A few years ago, I was on a mission to find a new fragrance. It was quite the ordeal and experiment for me as I tested many different ones. I ended up with a perfume by Coach called Poppy. I found I couldn't wear it very often, as my workplace is (as many are now) a "Fragrance Free" zone. Most hospitals and institutions are now "Fragrance Free" due to people's sensitivities and allergies. I hardly ever wore it. It ended up on my daughter's shelf. She has many different perfumes in her collection, and she is still collecting them as I write this.

I have noticed I am becoming very sensitive to strong scents, and I rarely wear any now. However, I make sure I am clean, and I wear deodorant every day. I would rather have no odour than a foul one. When I go out, sometimes I put on a small dab of something. It may even be a drop or two of essential oil such as lavender. This is another personal choice for each person. Please ensure when and if you wear perfume or cologne that it is not expired! Fragrances that are expired can change colour or start to smell bad, so make sure you go through them occasionally to get rid of the old bottles or samples in your collection.

Turn-offs include not only spoiled fragrances but bad breath. Halitosis can be a deal-breaker for some people. Keeping your teeth clean and breath fresh is very important for overall hygiene health. Breath sprays and mints are cheap and easy!

Human Touch

Rick Springfield said, "We all need the human touch." How you get yours is up to you. Going for a massage or getting a hair wash and haircut are other ways to get our needs met. Asking for a hug or holding someone's hand can help reinforce our connection to others in a non-sexual but intimate way. (By the way, I got a hug from Rick Springfield when I was 52 years old!)

Engaging in fun activities such as foreplay and flirting can make life more exciting. Get your Mojo on! Participating in sexual intercourse and other intimate activities such as kissing and touching have many health benefits. I invite you to do your research on the topic and decide what's right for you.

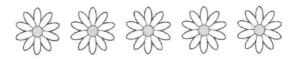

Sexual-Wellness Self-Assessment

On a scale of 1 to 4, 1 being very dissatisfied, 4 being very satisfied, where are you at in terms of satisfaction with your sexuality?

Circle one:

1 = Very dissatisfied. Horrible. Nonexistent.
2 = Dissatisfied. Not that great.
3 = Satisfied. It's okay.
4 = Very satisfied. Very content. Happy.

Sexual-Wellness Reflection

If you score on the bottom half of the scale, what can you do, moving forward, to improve your sexuality score? And when do you want to start making changes? How important is this to you? If you are scoring in the top half of the scale, what can you do to move toward a "four"?

Affirmations

- I am a sexual being.
- I am an attractive woman.
- I accept the sexual expression of others.
- I am free to express my sexuality.
- I accept my desire for sex and intimacy.
- It's okay if I don't want to have sex.
- I am open to trying out different ways to satisfy my sexual needs.
- I will talk to my doctor about my "privates" and sexual problems.
- I keep my sex life private, and that's okay.
- I respect my body and my choices.

Things to Try

- Write down what your feelings and thoughts are about sex and aging.
- Read articles and books about women, aging, and sex.
- Look at your naked body in the mirror, back, and front, and find three things you like about it.
- Tell your partner what you like in terms of intimacy and sex.
- Consider seeing a psychotherapist if you are not happy with your current sex life.
- Take a good look at yourself, and see if there is anything you could improve to enhance your attractiveness.
- Have a talk with your doctor about your sexual-health concerns.
- Take a pole-dancing class.

References

Kaplan, Helen Singer (1988). *The Illustrated Manual of Sex Therapy*, Second Edition. Routledge.

Kaplan, Helen Singer (1974). *The New Sex Therapy: Active Treatment of Sexual Dysfunctions*. Routledge.

Price, Joan (2014). *The Ultimate Guide to Sex After Fifty: How to Maintain — or Regain — a Spicy, Satisfying Sex Life.*

Sexuality Education Resource Centre Manitoba: serc.mb.ca

Chapter 8

Spiritual Wellness

You are not a human being having a spiritual experience—
you are a spiritual being having a human experience.

— Wayne Dyer

Body, mind, and soul—the triad of our existence as human beings. This chapter focuses on the "soul," otherwise known as the "inner you"—that place where our hidden feelings and thoughts are stored. When talking about total well-being and whole health, we often refer to the three main facets of the human experience. I believe having a soul is what makes us different from all other living creatures. Some may argue that dogs and other animals have a soul, and although I don't dispute that, I still think the soul of a dog and the soul of a person are two different things. The best way to describe the human soul is that invisible part of us that thinks, believes, dreams, and hopes. A person with an ailing soul would be empty, lost, and weary.

Another way to describe the human soul is "spirit." Spiritual wellness is having a sense of purpose in life and a value system. One of the assessment tools I use for screening for symptoms of depression asks, "Are you in good spirits most of the time?" This is the part of our being that is beyond the physical, beyond the obvious. You can't see the spirit, but you can sense it. It corresponds with our development and maturation. We grow into it as we question and explore. I believe the soul never dies. Our soul existed before we were born, and it will remain after the physical body is gone (hence the term "spirit world").

The spirit is the essence of what makes you individually unique. Your soul is at the root of your personality. It is your heart centre. (More on personality in the Emotional Wellness chapter.)

Understanding of spirit takes self-awareness and introspection. Being self-aware means asking ourselves questions about the state of our spirit: Do I feel connected to others? Do I like myself? Is there any hope for me? What brings me peace? Can I let go of things beyond my control? Am I comfortable with my beliefs about life and death? Do I know how to love? Have I been loved? Do I appreciate what is good in my life? Am I thankful? Do I practice an attitude of gratitude? What are my thoughts on violence? Is there a religious or other organization that can help me explore my spirituality?

My first exposure to spirituality was through religion. Religion was never a big thing in my home when I was growing up. When I was about eight or nine, I signed up for Sunday School at a local church. My parents didn't force me to go, nor did they discourage me. I learned about Jesus and won prizes for singing songs and reciting the Ten Commandments. I was proud to learn how to recite "The Lord's Prayer." This was my first real taste of organized religion. It was a fun experience for me, and I can still remember some of the songs we learned—*"Jesus loves me/this I know ..."* My parents never prayed or talked about God or Jesus. My mom said she was raised "Protestant," but I never really knew what that meant. I signed up for a summer bible camp when I was about 13. There was some more singing about Jesus and, most importantly, having fun with my newfound friends. I had a good experience with organized religion, although it wasn't much.

When I was in high school, I had a strange feeling come over me. It was like I had just "awakened" to my mortality. I wondered to myself, "Why am I here?" "What is the purpose of life?" My curiosity and inquisitiveness didn't go anywhere. I just knew I realized I had big questions with no answers at that point in my life.

As I matured, I learned more about God, the Universe, and how important it is to be kind to one another. I met my soon-to-be husband, who was Italian and came from a solid Catholic upbringing. Our relationship developed, our love grew, and to get married in a church, we felt it would be best if I got baptized in the Catholic faith. I went to catechism (Catholic school) and was baptized and confirmed as an adult. My future mother-in-law was a firm believer and was so pleased that I adopted the Catholic faith. I never had anything bad to say about Catholicism, but I started hearing disturbing things about it as time went on. Then I started hearing things about organized religion, in general, that didn't sit right with me. The "business" of the church meant that they would pass around a basket for donations at every mass to help keep the church going. Then I learned about the priests who abused children. And I heard stories about how the church condemned homosexuals and birth control. I could see how it turned some people off.

> Spirituality goes far beyond any form of organized religion. Be open to exploring this aspect of your life.

My spiritual journey has led me to a place of peace and comfort. I realize now that spirituality goes far beyond any form of organized religion. Spirituality is the quality of being concerned with beliefs and thoughts as opposed to material or physical things. The human spirit or soul is at the heart of spirituality. A person can be spiritual but not religious (SBNR). Some people find comfort in exploring different religions and perspectives, taking what fits and feels good, while leaving the rest. I have taken to visiting other churches. I am open to exploring a variety of faiths and practices.

Those who are "religious" may identify themselves as Christian, Catholic, or Protestant. They may say they attend the United Church, for example. Some may be Jewish and attend synagogue. Muslims worship in a mosque. Others may say they believe in God, but they are non-denominational. Buddhists have their own set of beliefs and may or may not go to a temple to practice worship. Hindus may attend a temple, or they may have a shrine in their own home. There are many world religions based on cultures and traditions going back thousands of years. Non-believers (people who don't believe in God) identify themselves as atheist. Those who are not sure if there is a God are agnostic.

The Seven Sacred Teachings of the Indigenous peoples pass along stories to learn about morals and spirituality. Those seven teachings are Wisdom (Beaver), Bravery/Courage (Bear), Honesty (Sabe a.k.a. Sasquatch), Respect (Buffalo), Truth (Turtle), Humility (Wolf), Love (Eagle). These wonderful stories help us learn about the depths of our human spirit and how we can live in harmony with each other and our communities.

No matter what your beliefs, thoughts, or feelings are on the spiritual aspects of life, the main thing is that we respect and appreciate each other's differences. I would hope we could all agree one of our most common human needs is the need to feel loved. Self-love comes first, because if we don't love ourselves, we may have trouble loving others. Teaching self-love at a young age is paramount— any religion or doctrine that doesn't teach this is doing its people a disservice. To feel loved by others means we need to give love to each other. If there was more love in this world, there would be more peace and less suffering.

When we experience self-love (and I mean in the most profound sense, not ego-driven greed and selfishness), we can fully experience and apply what is called "The Golden Rule." This is a moral ideal that can be utilized in our relationships with each other—not only personally, but in our communities, countries, and the world. The Golden Rule teaches us tolerance and acceptance of different cultures and religions, encouraging peace and kindness. Many world religions teach a version of this concept. The Christian version of this is, "Do to others as you have them do to you." In Hinduism, they say, "Do not do to others what would cause pain if done to you." The Judaism belief says, "What is hateful to you, do not do to your neighbour. This is the whole Torah; all the rest is commentary." One of my favourites comes from Confucianism— "One word which sums up the basis of all good conduct ... loving-kindness. Do not do to others what you do not want to be done to yourself." Be good, do good.

There are many ways we can exercise, practice, and develop spirituality. Many of these practices and ideas can help us connect with our heart centre and our "soul." Pick and choose what works for you.

Spiritual practices include:

1. Prayer
2. Recite mantras (motivating words or phrases)
3. Practice mindfulness (Live in the moment, the Power of Now)
4. Meditate
5. Create a mandala to help you gain knowledge from within
6. Practice loving-kindness
7. Practice forgiveness
8. Express gratitude
9. Be aware of abundance in your life
10. Live joyfully
11. Pay it forward
12. Attend sacred services
13. Watch services online, TV, radio
14. Read the sacred texts such as the Torah, the Christian Bible, the Quran, or the Vedas
15. Find a talisman, inspirational coin, or rock to hold or keep in your pocket (e.g., I have a smooth rock that says "Faith" on it)
16. Visit a store that sells religious and spiritual items; browse through, and see what stands out to you
17. Chakra balancing
18. Make a vision board
19. Wear jewelry that is an outward symbol of your faith (e.g., I have a necklace with a cross on it, and a rosary bracelet I had blessed by a Catholic priest)
20. Immerse yourself in nature—Japanese "Forest bathing"
21. Walk a labyrinth
22. Honour and activate your inner goddess
23. Experience a sense of feeling grounded, e.g., try bare feet in the grass
24. Be still
25. Engage in self-reflection
26. Do deep breathing
27. Practice yoga
28. Enjoy the wonder of serendipity and synchronicity
29. Allow yourself to reflect on your spiritual intuition, such as dreams, messages, visions, or other signs. Consider these as awareness tools of spirituality—perhaps ways to connect to, and communicate with, your higher self

30. Consider being open to having an "angel" or "spirit guide" to help you find strength and direction
31. Journal
32. Speak with Spiritual Health Practitioners or those who are open-minded regarding speaking about their religion, beliefs, non-beliefs, and spirituality
33. Release the need for high expectations—go with the flow of natural rhythms, and surrender to it

We are all on the path of spiritual enlightenment. Some of us don't even realize it. Becoming aware of our spiritual needs is part of our "awakening." When we realize we are mortal souls—our life on Earth is finite—it changes us. The full comprehension of our situation helps give us meaning, purpose, power, and intention. We are more aware of actions and inactions and how we see others in this world. We may become more religious or feel closer to God. We may pray or partake in rituals.

Aging is a staircase—the upward ascension of the human spirit, bringing us into wisdom, wholeness and authenticity. As you may know, the entire world operates on a universal law: entropy, the second law of thermodynamics. Entropy means everything in the world—everything—is in a state of decline and decay, the arch. There's only one exception to this universal law, and that is the human spirit, which can continue to evolve upwards.

— Jane Fonda

For those who don't believe in God, they may believe in the "Big Bang" and how we are all part of an intricate and spectacular cosmic experiment. "Source," "The Universe," "Higher Power," "Creator," "Maker," and "Great Being" are other terms people may use to describe the force outside of themselves. Others say connecting to nature makes them feel more at peace. Some find comfort in discovering we are all connected—we are all energy—the trees, the earth, and each other.

Our belief in karma, knowing that the energy we put out, either good or bad, comes back to us tenfold, can help keep us kind and compassionate. Knowing that suffering is part of the human experience can help us appreciate and enjoy those special and joyful moments all the more.

Mindfulness and meditation may be part of our spiritual practice. Quieting our minds and listening to the soul of who we are helps us feel more grounded and relaxed. There are many other terms and approaches to describe our relationship to the world, the universe, and each other. We can learn from the teachings of thought leaders on spirituality such as Wayne Dyer, Eckhart Tolle, Louise Hay, and Marianne Williamson.

Our spiritual wellness depends on how comfortable we are with our "be"-ing. Tapping into our higher consciousness and self-awareness is achieved through introspection and contemplation. Curiosity and openness to the divine is a magical and mystical experience. If we are confident in the approach we take to understand our lives, our connections, the meaning of life, our purpose, leaving a legacy, and what happens to us when we die, we may say that we have a healthy level of spiritual wellness.

If we feel we don't know what to believe, we feel our God has forsaken us, we feel lost, or we don't have a life purpose, then we would have a low spiritual wellness level. Perhaps we have our beliefs, but we are "non-practicing." If we are comfortable and satisfied with our choices and behaviour, that would be considered favourable spiritual wellness. I invite you to take the next step in deepening your relationship with your heart centre and spiritual enlightenment.

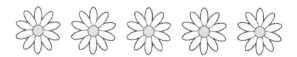

Spiritual-Wellness Self-Assessment

On a scale of 1 to 4, 1 being very dissatisfied, 4 being very satisfied, where are you at in terms of satisfaction with your spirituality?

Circle one:

1 = Very dissatisfied. Horrible. Nonexistent.
2 = Dissatisfied. Not that great.
3 = Satisfied. It's okay.
4 = Very satisfied. Very content. Happy.

Spiritual-Wellness Reflection

If you score on the bottom half of the scale, what can you do, moving forward, to improve your Spiritual-Wellness score? And when do you want to start making changes? How important is this to you? If you are scoring in the top half of the scale, what can you do to move toward a "four"?

Affirmations

- I am open to enhancing my spiritual wellness.
- I give love freely.
- I take time to be quiet.
- I have meaning in my day-to-day life.
- I honour my hopes, dreams, and aspirations.
- My curiosity enables me to learn about others' spiritual beliefs.
- I am becoming aware of meaning and purpose in my life.
- I am in touch with my heart centre.
- I practice loving-kindness daily.
- My spiritual needs are being met.
- I actively pursue activities that bring me closer to nature.
- I take time for myself every day.
- I love myself.
- I am at peace and feel contentment.

Things to Try

- Have an open discussion with someone about what their beliefs are.
- Visit a church or other gathering place, and pray to your God or your higher self.
- Do something for yourself.
- Write down how you view your spirituality.
- Take a walk in nature (have a "forest bath"), and notice the small things.
- Take three deep breaths when you need to slow down.
- Every day, write down three things you are grateful for.
- Download an app to help with mindfulness, meditation, or other related topics.

References

The Golden Rule Poster, Pflaum Publishing Group (2000).

Strout, K. A. & Howard, E. P. (2015). Five Dimensions of Wellness and Predictor of Cognitive Health Protection in Community-Dwelling Older Adults. A Historical COLLAGE Cohort Study. *Journal of Holistic Nursing* 33(1), 6-18.

Chapter 9

Environmental Wellness

We are what we see. We are products of our surroundings.

— Amber Valletta

How well is your world? When we live in a "sick" environment or aren't treating it with care, we will ultimately feel the effects. When our living spaces and communities are considered healthy, we stand a better chance of feeling well while in them.

Our environment can be as small as our bedroom or office at work, or it can be further reaching, such as our home or neighbourhood. Our workplace could also be our home. Our communities are the environments we live, play, and work in. Living in a clean and hygienically sound home can help us feel good about ourselves. It can help ward off illnesses. Having healthy air in our house or workplace is key to having healthy lungs. Living close to a busy street (e.g., the freeway) can cause long-term health issues because of the increased pollution. Smoke in the air, whether it is firsthand or secondhand, can cause lung diseases such as cancer. Asbestos that's hiding in our buildings can also cause cancer (mesothelioma). Black mold (or any colour!) can make us sick. Mold can flourish if the conditions are just right (it loves damp and dark). Bug or rodent infestations are horrible. Mice can cause a viral lung disease (Hantavirus Pulmonary Syndrome). On the flip side, there are benefits to living in an environment with lots of natural light. The more windows, the better, and there are considerations for what direction your windows face (e.g., East view for sunrise, West view for sunsets).

Consider who or what we share our living space with: The three Ps—People, Pets, and Plants. Are you living with someone else such as a friend or a significant other? Do you have a roommate? Do you live with family? Hopefully, the people you live with are kind, respectful, and helpful. If we don't have amenable spouses or housemates, this can make for a stressful environment. If you don't live with anybody, are you okay with that? Perhaps you prefer to live alone. Maybe you would consider having someone move in with you, or you want to move in with someone else. Pets can enhance our homes and provide companionship and "someone" to care for. Dogs and cats are two of the most popular pets, and a dog can feel like a family member! I don't have a green thumb when it comes to indoor plants, but if you are, enjoy the greenery and caring for your plants. I know of many older people who love looking after their indoor plants and flowers. Warmer weather can also provide opportunities for flower or vegetable gardening. Bringing the outdoors indoors can add a special touch to our environments.

"Raising awareness on the most pressing environmental issues of our time is more important than ever." — Leonardo DiCaprio

Climate Change (Global Warming) is a real concern, and the global response to this crisis has been mixed. Although scientists and environmental activists like Greta Thunberg, from Sweden, are sounding the alarm, it just seems like people aren't doing enough to "save our planet." World leaders, politicians, policy-makers, business owners, and the general public need to be educated and work together to make positive changes. The future looks bright, with plans to use renewable energy sources such as solar and wind power. Electric cars are here, and who knows what the future will bring!

We can each do our part in reducing our carbon emissions. For example, my husband, Agapito, has been riding his bike to the hospital where he works almost every day for the past 30 years (and counting!). He says there are so many benefits, including reducing fuel emissions, saving gas money, saving on parking, keeping physically fit, and getting fresh air and sunshine. Sometimes he even saves time getting home when there are traffic problems.

There are things within our control for taking care of our environment. Consider your role in supporting an eco-friendly lifestyle. Reducing waste can help keep garbage out of our landfills. Reusing items can help prevent the manufacturing of more products, and it can help save money. Refuse to buy things that have lots of packaging—buy in bulk if you can. Repair things that break instead of tossing them out and buying new. Buy used to save money and the environment. Recycling wherever and whenever possible shows that we care about our precious land and environment. Composting "greens" and "browns" can help put nutrient-rich waste back into the soil, where it belongs. Choose non-toxic cleaning products or those that have all natural ingredients. Read labels and see what chemicals you are using, and research to see if they are okay for the environment (or your body!) Putting trash where it belongs, instead of littering, demonstrates a sense of pride and good manners. Who wants to see your garbage on the side of the road? Cutting back on the use of plastics is good for our precious oceans.

Put a colourful display of flowers in a vase in your home or office. It will add vibrancy and a bit of nature to your environment.

You could play relaxing music (piano or acoustic is nice) and light some fragranced candles to enhance your home. If using scents, go for the authentic and natural ones. My favourite essential oils are eucalyptus, peppermint, orange, lavender, and lemongrass. For candles, stick to beeswax or soy. If you have a dimmer switch, turn down the lights when talking with someone or listening to music. Himalayan salt lamps are soothing and relaxing. You could also look into the art of Feng Shui, which could give you some ideas on where to place objects and furniture, with particular attention to the "flow of energy." Textures such as soft pillows, fuzzy blankets, or hardwood floors could also add ambiance and warmth, giving you a homey feel. The scents from flowers, a wood fire, and baking can also provide comfort. Opening windows or window coverings adds fresh air and sunlight. Decorate your home for the changing seasons or holidays.

When you look at your home and belongings, do you find them in an orderly fashion, or are things everywhere? Is there a place for everything, and is everything in its place? If you find there is too much stuff and too much clutter, perhaps it's time to go through and reduce the number of things you own. Hoarding is a serious mental-health problem that results in living spaces being overcrowded, leading to issues such as tripping and fire hazards. I know when I declutter, I feel terrific. Letting go of things I no longer need is uplifting. It's as though a weight has been lifted off my shoulders. Too much stuff can weigh a person down. It seems like we spend the first 50 years accumulating stuff and the next 50 years disposing of it!

> Instead of asking for a gift you don't really need, consider replacing something you already have. Upgrading can be awesome, too.

Of all the older adults I have worked with, I would say the majority of them, in their later years, end up living in one small room or apartment. Some are in nursing homes or studio apartments. There isn't room for too much stuff, so it's a good idea to start condensing so your kids or relatives don't have to help you go through it all one day. If you haven't looked into what minimalist living is, you may want to check it out!

I adopted a tidying exercise by Marie Kondo called the KonMari method. She teaches that, when we want to purge unwanted or useless items, try holding the item. If it brings you a feeling of joy,

128

keep it. If it doesn't bring joy, thank it for its service and then discard it. Discard could mean giving it away, donating it, recycling it, or throwing it away. If the item doesn't give joy but has a useful purpose, you should keep it. I have gotten rid of many items by using KonMari. It works great. The end result is an environment of things that bring me joy. I am then surrounded by things that are beautiful, familiar, and useful.

Our household environment should be age-friendly. "Universal Design" is a concept applied to environments that are usable and enjoyed by everyone, no matter what their abilities or limitations.

If you want to clean out the items hanging in your closet, but you are not sure what to get rid of, turn all the hangers backward. As you use the items, turn the hangers forward. In a year (or after several months of going through all the seasons), you will discover what items you don't use, and then you can decide which to discard.

"Visitability" is enhanced when there are no stairs to get through the main doors. There should be ease of access for people who are using canes, walkers, or wheelchairs. It is a bonus if we can adapt our homes so we can "age in place." To stay in our houses for a longer time, we may need to add a chair lift to get upstairs to the bedroom or convert our bathroom to include a walk-in bathtub with a low step-in. Adding safety rails or grab bars in the shower or a raised toilet seat can help us manage more independently. Subscribing to a personal-alarm device with an auto-alert fall-detection option can also provide peace of mind to ourselves and our loved ones. For more information, check out aginginplace.org.

As we get older, we may find a need to downsize and move. We may move from a house to a condominium. Or from a condominium to an apartment. Or from a two-bedroom apartment to a one-bedroom apartment. Perhaps we are moving from our daughter's home into a nursing home. Maybe you are moving to an assisted-living residence with your sibling. No matter what precipitated the move (finances, health, other), downsizing is often an overwhelming task. That's why it's important to declutter and minimize as we get older. Instead of accumulating items, it is suggested we sell, give away, or donate things. The more we do this ahead of time, the easier it will be on our relatives down the line.

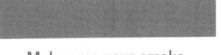

Make sure your smoke detectors and carbon-monoxide detectors are in good working order!

Another essential wellness feature of our environment is how safe we feel in it. Do we think we can walk in the neighbourhood and feel safe? Is there a police presence that feels reassuring and comforting? Some communities feel safer than others. Gated communities offer peace of mind. Seniors' apartment blocks usually have safety features such as a locked front door, warning "Do not let people in that you don't know." Fostering good relationships with our neighbours can also help us feel protected, and just knowing someone is there if we need them is reassuring. For those of us who live alone, this is particularly helpful. Having good deadbolts on the doors and an alarm system can also help us feel safe and secure.

The health of our environment directly affects our well-being. We have control of how we want our environment to look and feel. Being surrounded by nature and simply hearing bird calls can help reduce stress. Keeping our environment clean, safe, clutter-free, and beautiful will enhance our outlook and overall wellness.

Environmental-Wellness Self-Assessment

On a scale of 1 to 4, 1 being very dissatisfied, 4 being very satisfied, where are you at in terms of satisfaction with your environment?

Circle one:

1 = Very dissatisfied. Horrible. Nonexistent.
2 = Dissatisfied. Not that great.
3 = Satisfied. It's okay.
4 = Very satisfied. Very content. Happy.

Environmental-Wellness Reflection

If you score on the bottom half of the scale, what can you do, moving forward, to improve your environment? And when do you want to start making changes? How important is this to you? If you are scoring in the top half of the scale, what can you do to move toward a "four"?

Affirmations

- My home is healthy and happy.
- I like my housemates, and they respect me.
- I love my pets; they make me feel loved and give me joy.
- I love the positive vibes at my workplace.
- I enjoy walking around my neighbourhood.
- I feel safe in my community.
- The air I breathe is clean and purifying.
- I am decluttering as I go.
- I am not accumulating any more things, just replacing them as needed.

- I will swap, trade, or barter for items I need to help reduce the amount of "stuff" in the world.
- I have good neighbours, and I practice respectful conduct.
- I take Climate Change seriously, and I want to do what I can to help.

Things to Try

- Read up on or watch Marie Kondo, and try to clean up a section of your home.
- If you don't feel safe in your current neighbourhood, consider moving or talking to your neighbours about a "Neighbourhood Watch" program.
- Next time you are baking, deliver some treats to your next-door neighbour.
- Consider getting a pet or, at the very least, pet-sitting for someone.
- When your neighbours are outside, say, "Hello! How are you?"
- Whenever you buy a new piece of clothing, try to eliminate two items in your closet or dresser you no longer wear or use.
- When you see litter on the sidewalk or road, pick it up, and dispose of it.
- Recycle wherever and whenever possible.
- Learn about composting, and get a composter and a small compost bin.
- Read up on Climate Change, and find out what you can do to reduce your carbon footprint (start with transportation, power, food supply, and stuff we buy).

Chapter 10

Recreational Wellness

Sometimes, the inessential is essential.

— T.L. Rese

Having fun and pursuing recreational activities are integral parts of a balanced lifestyle. Too much work and no play make for a dull, boring life. Doing something enjoyable is also a good stress reducer. Remember when we were little kids, and everything was fun? Children know how to laugh—that's for sure. How come we don't laugh as much as kids do?

Enjoyable recreation and leisure activities are hard to come by if you are too busy to make time for them. There was a point in my life where I realized I wasn't having any fun. Everything was work, work, work, and too many responsibilities. I had to make a concerted effort to schedule playtime. Hobbies and leisure activities can be sedentary, active, social, or solitary.

Here are some examples of recreational activities:

1. Arts and crafts—Crafting, writing, calligraphy, photography, knitting, sewing, quilting, drawing, colouring (check out adult colouring books!), painting, card-making, scrapbooking, baking, cooking, jigsaw puzzles, carving, beading, pottery, making jewelry

2. Genealogy—Groups, Individual hobby, DNA tests, Family Tree, Family History, Ancestry

3. Collections—Stamps, dolls, coins, *Star Wars*, frogs, shells

4. Reading—Paperbacks, hardcovers, magazines, ebooks, audiobooks. Available in libraries, bookstores, thrift shops, and online stores (new and used) such as Amazon, Abe Books

5. Word and math games—crosswords, word search, Sudoku, Scrabble

6. Entertainment—Radio, television, online videos, internet, movie and T.V. show streaming services (such as Netflix— beware of getting caught up in binge-watching or Netflix marathons!), social media, theatre, symphony, movies, opera, ballet, comedy, concerts, shopping, parades, fairs, trade shows

7. Gaming—Casinos, online gambling, games you can play on your phone such as "Candy Crush," video games, bingo, escape games, board games, card games

8. Travel—Traveling within your own state, province, or country, or beyond; listening to or watching travel documentaries or travelogues

9. Seasonal Activities—Going to your cottage (or renting one), camping, taking R.V. or travel-trailer trips

10. Outdoors—Hiking, bird watching, geocaching (outdoor treasure hunting with GPS-enabled devices), swimming, walking, cycling, running, horseback riding, mountain climbing, gardening (indoor gardening, too!), picking wildflowers, berry picking, mushroom picking, fishing, hunting, trapping, boating, spending time by the beach, farming, shopping at farmer's markets

11. Winter—Snowshoeing, cross-country skiing, downhill skiing, skating, snowshoeing, sledding, tobogganing, curling

12. Socializing—Going out for dinner or drinks, having friends over to play games, going out for a meal or planning a meal to have at home with friends, attending women's retreats, enjoying pajama parties, looking after children (grandchildren), visiting older relatives or friends, joining a seniors' group

13. Sports—Watching or participating in sports, hockey, tennis, baseball, pickleball, or lawn bowling

14. Music—Listening to music, playing (or learning to play) a musical instrument, joining a choir, singing, enjoying digital music-streaming services (such as Spotify or Apple Music)

15. Podcasts—Listening to digital audio files on an electronic device (usually pre-recorded episodes that are part of a series)

16. Art—Drawing, painting, visiting art galleries or museums

17. Learning—Learning a new skill such as flower arranging, woodworking, flying a plane, or learning a new language

18. Physical Activity—Swimming, Zumba, golfing, bowling, walking, martial arts, barre fitness (using a ballet barre), doing aerobics

19. Dancing—Taking dance lessons, moving to music, line dancing, square dancing, tango, rumba, or belly dancing

20. Relaxation—Napping, meditating, getting a massage, indulging in a spa day, getting a manicure and/or pedicure,

napping in a hammock, watching the sunrise or sunset, stargazing, cloud watching, sitting on a patio swing listening to the birds

21. Home improvement—Decorating, renovating, rearranging furniture, painting walls, replacing flooring

22. Activism such as Animal Rights or Environmental— Participating in Animal Rescue, visiting Animal Shelters, supporting Greenpeace, People for the Ethical Treatment of Animals (PETA), Stop the Spray (to end non-essential herbicide spraying in the public forests)

23. Volunteering—Helping out at a local food or animal shelter, serving as a hospital gift-shop clerk, providing telephone support to caregivers, visiting people in nursing homes or visiting hospice patients

Hold a "Fun-Raiser"—
a party just for fun!

We have to balance working and taking care of our responsibilities with leisure and fun in our lives. If we spend too much time on recreation and having fun, then other areas of our lives can suffer. Too much gambling can lead to money problems. Too much TV or time on screens can lead to a sedentary lifestyle, which comes with health risks.

Laughter is the best medicine. Giggling, smiling, rolling-on-the-floor laughter is a good stress reliever. Laughing with family or friends is even more fun. Laughing so hard that you pee your pants is even better! Going to see a funny movie or sharing a humorous video or joke can help lift a person's mood. It doesn't take much these days to find humour. It's everywhere. Some of my favourite people who make me laugh include author Sophie Kinsella (the *Shopaholic* series) and Loretta Laroche, author of *Juicy Aging, Juicy Aging*. There's even a thing called Laughter Yoga. Seek it, and ye shall find it.

Pets can keep us entertained as well. Taking the time to learn about different dog breeds, talking to people about important factors to consider in a dog (e.g., shedding vs. non-shedding; small, medium, or large) can become a big project. Consider the costs such as vet visits, grooming, training, food, licensing, crate/aquarium/beds. Visiting shelters or breeders can help you decide what kind of dog or cat you want. Rescuing a dog or cat can also be a rewarding experience.

Research other types of pets, and find out how much they cost, what their needs are, and what fits into your lifestyle. Some people prefer "show dogs," and some become "breeders." Others prefer a cat or a bird. I know of people who have had pets such as snakes, lizards, and hedgehogs! When I was very young, my first pet was a turtle! The excitement builds up until the day your new pet comes home.

If you have the time, it's also possible to combine your desire to help others out by joining a cause to raise funds. Some ideas that come to mind are the annual "walks," "runs," or "cycles" that you can sign up for (e.g., "Run for the Cure"). You can get some exercise and raise money for a good cause at the same time.

In 2019, I participated in the "Skate Your Butt Off" event in California that raised money for the Anal Cancer Foundation. We roller skated on a pop-up roller rink outdoors. Other people like to register for marathons or triathlons (just for themselves, not for fundraising), and these are held all over the world. In 2019, the winner of the Boston Marathon received $150,000 USD cash! These events can take you to places you've never been before.

Go to the people and the places
that set a spark in your soul.

— Anonymous

If you are a person who likes to travel, how do you choose where you want to go? Do you go by where other people have been? Do you have specific places you want to go one day (a travel bucket list of sorts)? I was talking to a 79-year-old woman who showed me a large world map on her wall. She and her husband put a small dot on the locations they had travelled to. There were dots all over the map! There must have been more than 100. They tried to travel at least twice a year. I asked her, "What is your most favourite place in the world that you have visited?" She said, without any hesitancy, "Bali, Indonesia." At that moment, I realized my brother-in-law had said Bali was one of his favourite places, and I also remembered I'd read about it in *Eat, Pray, Love*. I decided to put this on my list of travel destinations. I tend to pick popular locations that others say are good.

I love to travel. One of my rules is that I have to try something new every time I go to a new place—even if it's something that scares me. My husband and I went to Costa Rica (to an all-inclusive resort) and planned to go zip lining. This was something that scared me because it felt dangerous. I am not a risk-taker, so this was a big deal for me. Although I was nervous about doing it, once we got strapped in and I saw everyone else excited to do it, I started to feel excited, too. The event organizers were very good, and I had a lot of fun soaring over the rain forest!

Some of my favourite trips have been to warm places where we could spend time on a beach. There are lots of fun things to do on or around the water. I have learned how to do things like "rock hop," "whale watch," and "boogie board." "Shelling" is a beach activity that includes looking for cool shells, walking on the beach, and sometimes you can even find some sea glass or a sand dollar. I have been blessed with seeing sea turtles and being close to one while swimming in "Turtle Cove." Another time my husband and I decided to go to a nude beach! We got naked—what a thrill!

In the summer, freshwater lakes are sprinkled with boaters; sometimes they are pulling water skiers or tubes behind with laughing, screeching people in tow. Sailboating, paddleboarding, and windsurfing take some skill. Floating around on an inner tube or an inflatable floating lounge chair can offer relaxation.

Thrill-seekers love to do things that scare them. Think of the feeling you get when you are on a roller coaster. It may make you so afraid that you don't want to go on it. The feeling of being tossed about and the fear that you may fall out may hold you back. Or perhaps you are afraid you will get sick. Doing something for the thrill of it can make you feel alive. My friend Maureen (my "Crazy-Shit Friend," as termed by Miriam Castilla) and I went zip lining at a local corn maze, and there was a 60-foot drop at the end. I didn't think I could do it. It was like walking the plank off a ship. I watched my friend and the others in the group do it, and they all encouraged me. It was either that, or I'd have to walk down the stairs. So, I got strapped in, and I was attached to a bungee-like cord. The guy told me, "Just walk like normal. Don't think about it too much." Before I knew it, I was dropping down. It was exhilarating! I am so glad I did it.

Each time I do something that scares me, it makes me feel a little more confident. I don't know if I could ever do a full-on bungee jump, or tandem skydive, but you never know! I do have an interest in going parasailing, though. Hopefully, one day!

When you are enjoying an activity, you may notice how time goes so quickly. Before you know it, an hour or two has flown by. Sometimes when I am writing, I don't realize how much time has gone by. Meaningful and pleasurable activities can help you get into the "flow." "Flow" makes people happy. If your work doesn't give you "flow," perhaps you can find it in hobbies or other non-work-related activities. Maybe you or someone you know has spent hours painting, reading, or watching sports. Those can create "flow."

Some people make a living helping others have fun and pursue recreational activities. They are called Recreational Therapists. These therapists are allied healthcare professionals who work with people of all ages. Most nursing homes, hospitals, and other residences have recreational therapists who provide an assessment of individuals and determine their interests and abilities. In particular, the long-term care industry knows the importance of having fun! When you are retired, and others are making your meals and cleaning your clothes, there is nothing left to do but fill your time with your interests and hobbies. Whether it's in person, on the phone, or a video call, family visits become very important to those in nursing homes. It could be the highlight of their day!

The pursuit of hobbies, recreation, and leisurely interests provides many benefits. It can be combined with socialization, relaxation, stress-reduction, and physical activity. There is fun to be had for people of any age. Excitement, happiness, peace-of-mind, distraction, and relaxation are great benefits of your feel-good activity choices.

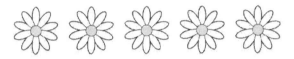

Recreational-Wellness Self-Assessment

On a scale of 1 to 4, 1 being very dissatisfied, 4 being very satisfied, where are you at in terms of satisfaction with your recreational habits?

Circle one:

1 = Very dissatisfied. Horrible. Nonexistent.
2 = Dissatisfied. Not that great.
3 = Satisfied. It's okay.
4 = Very satisfied. Very content. Happy.

Recreational-Wellness Reflection

If you score on the bottom half of the scale, what can you do, moving forward, to improve your Recreational-Wellness score? And when do you want to start making changes? How important is this to you? If you are scoring in the top half of the scale, what can you do to move toward a "four"?

Affirmations

- I make sure I laugh every day.
- I love to have fun.
- I look for fun opportunities.
- I will relax and enjoy my free time.
- I enjoy playing games.
- I like to spend my leisure time alone.
- I enjoy doing things that are fun and get me moving.
- I will do something that scares me.

Things to Try

- Do something that scares you.
- Make time to schedule some fun.
- Plan a dinner date with friends.
- Go camping.
- Plan a hike somewhere you've never been.
- Take photos and make an album.
- Buy a new board game, and play with friends.
- Read a book you've been waiting to dig in to.
- Download an app that is fun or relaxing (e.g., colouring, games).
- Do some word-search puzzles.
- Plan a trip, and do something exciting.
- Plan a trip, and relax.
- Listen to some music that matches your mood (e.g., fun, relaxing, cool), or try listening to a type of music you've never listened to before.

Chapter 11

Financial Wellness

Financial wellness is the state of living in which your well-being is measured by the quality of your life, not just wealth.

— Jason Vitug, B.S. (Finance), M.B.A.

What about health, wealth, and happiness? Isn't that what we wish for everyone? "Wealth" is a subjective term. What makes one person feel "wealthy" may not be enough for the next person. Happiness research from Purdue University in the USA tells us that, if you make at least $75,000 USD per year, then you won't be much happier if you make more than that. We often think if we had more money, we'd be happier, but that's not always the case.

Financial wellness means having enough money to meet your needs. Having enough income or savings to help pay for safe and comfortable living conditions is one of our primary needs. There are food requirements, paying for utilities such as heat and water, transportation, medications, healthcare, clothing, and other essentials such as soap and towels. If you have enough money for these daily essentials, you are in an excellent position.

There are many other financial-related considerations to think about. For example, did you think about (or were you able to think about) putting money away for retirement? For those who work, your employer may have a retirement pension plan they contribute to. My employer pays into a pension, and so do I.

On the financial-legal side, some documents can be prepared to help ensure your assets are protected. A Power of Attorney (P.O.A.) document can be prepared to help ensure that, if you were unable to act on your behalf, someone you trust has been legally appointed to take care of your affairs. Preparing a Last Will and Testament is also an important piece of financial planning, especially if you have assets to go to specific people or organizations. The Will and P.O.A.

BEWARE OF SCAMMERS

My mother told me a story about when my grandmother hired a random guy who had an ad in the newspaper. She needed someone to install her new carpet in the living room and dining room. Two men and a woman came in and installed the carpet. She paid cash. Then my grandmother wanted some new carpet for her bedroom, so they went into the bedroom to measure. She prepaid, $500 cash, for the rose-coloured carpet they were to order and install at a later date. They left and never came back. She had no way to get in touch with them, as the number in the newspaper had been disconnected. Then she discovered that some of her gold jewelry was missing.

My grandmother had been robbed. She thought it would be better to hire a stranger who charged less than someone reputable and trustworthy that she knew. Moving forward, my grandmother said, "Never hire someone random you find in the newspaper." Be very careful if you are hiring a handyman. Make sure you have references and contact information.

---

are often prepared at the same time. An Enduring (or Durable) P.O.A. is especially important to consider, as it will take effect if you are unable to speak or act on your own behalf due to an illness or injury such as a stroke, dementia, or a traumatic brain injury.

Safeguarding your money and assets is an essential key to financial wellness. There are many scammers out there who will try to trick you out of handing over your money. These scam artists can intrude via telephone, email, your front door, or text messages.

Sometimes people are scammed due to poor decision-making and naivety, leading them to lose hundreds or even thousands of dollars. For example, you may require some repairs on your home, such as a new window, and you call a company that you think is reputable, but it ends up they are not. And how many calls have we received that say, "You have won ... just give us your credit-card number so we can send you your gift". Or an email that says, "You have inherited five million dollars . . . just provide us with your name, address, and banking information, and we will transfer the money to your account."

We need to be aware of the latest scams and know how to ignore them or report them. I have learned, if someone calls me to say they are going to help me get rid of the virus on my computer that they have discovered, to keep them on the line as long as possible without giving them any of my personal information. The longer I keep them on the line, the less time they will have to try and scam someone else.

Donations to charity and other causes you believe in can help you feel good. Often a receipt can be used for tax purposes. The donations you make can be claimed at year end, and you can get a little tax break because of it. Whether it's a one-time donation on "Giving Tuesday," your yearly contribution to the "Heart and Stroke Foundation" or "Alzheimer Society," or a monthly transfer of funds to your local church, these may qualify for a tax benefit. Tax laws are always changing, so if you're not sure, it's a good idea to check with your charities or a reputable accountant. (It's also interesting to note here that T.V. ministries and local ministries tend to appeal to the charitable nature of older people for donations.)

When it comes to being taken advantage of financially, it seems like family members are the worst. I have heard of many situations where an older mother gives money to her adult son so that he can continue to feed his addiction, problem-gambling, or excessive spending habits. What starts as a caring motherly (or parental) duty slowly leads to the mother not having enough money to pay for her own needs. This is particularly true when the mother (divorced or widowed) and son live together, and the son has never moved out of the home. There is a common phenomenon in my line of work called "Son in basement." We need to be on the lookout for what *seems* to be a mutually beneficial arrangement, but underneath, it is not. If you or someone you know is in this kind of situation, reach out to a friend or other trusted professional for advice on dealing with it.

One way to avoid the need for Power of Attorney (P.O.A.) and other legal counsel is to have someone you trust named as a joint account holder on your bank account(s). That way, if you were ever unable to get to the bank (or if you died), that person would be able to access the funds without the need for a lawyer. The other thing you can do is, if you own a house or other property, or you have more considerable assets, you can add this trusted person to the title(s). Also, make sure someone else you trust has the keys to your home and vehicle. The same thing goes for investments and other financial matters. When asked for a "beneficiary," make sure you name someone so that those things are taken care of.

There are many ways to get an income, and for some, that means help from the government. If you are working and making enough to make ends meet, that's great. If you are in a two-income household, hopefully, you are in an even-better position. If you are not working, you can apply for financial aid. For those who retire, there is often a pension or other retirement income to provide for a comfortable living situation.

If your income is such that you can't afford the home of your dreams or the one-bedroom apartment you always wanted, there are "rent-geared-to-income" apartments that you can apply for. A "reverse mortgage" is another way to get income if you are older and own a home. Moving in with a family member or friend is also an option, in which you pay a monthly rental fee for room and board. If you are considering moving in with someone or having someone move in with you, it's always a good idea to have a legal document written up by an attorney (or at least a written agreement that both parties review, agree to, and sign). You never know when and if things can backfire. There is information on "Roommate," "Lease," or "Rental" Agreements on the internet to help you decide what is the right document for your situation.

Debt can be a significant burden for some people. Most credit-card companies happily give people credit with a hefty interest charge and minimum monthly payment requirements. Mortgages on a new home can be for hundreds of thousands of dollars and can span 30 years or longer. These hefty bi-weekly or monthly payments can become burdensome if you lose part of your income or if some other financial emergency or expenditure comes along.

Buying or leasing a new car can also get you locked into bi-weekly or monthly payments. Sometimes the 0% financing is hard to resist. Lines of Credit are handy to have, but these and other bank loans come with an interest charge that can also add up. If you find yourself in a situation where your debt is too high, and your income is too low, it may benefit you to sit down with an accountant or other financial professional to sort out how you will get your debt under control. Not having money to spend on the things you value and treasure most can be a real downer, and debit or credit counselling can get you moving in the right direction.

Deciding on the right time to retire is a big decision for many people. For those who have worked for 20-30 years or more, the consideration is often related to finances. In Canada, there are government programs that folks can apply for or are eligible for. The Canada Pension Plan (C.P.P.), Old Age Security (O.A.S.), and Guaranteed Income Supplement (G.I.S.) are the three primary sources of income for older Canadians. The C.P.P. can be applied for as early as age 60, and the O.A.S. and G.I.S. kick into effect at age 65. O.A.S. is available to all Canadians, no matter their income. The G.I.S. is available only to those who need a little top-up because they don't have substantial retirement pension income.

Related to financial well-being is insurance. It seems that if you don't have insurance, you will be sorry you don't. And if you do have it, you won't need it. There are all kinds of insurance options. The main ones that I am aware of are Extended Health Coverage, Disability Insurance, Life Insurance, Car Insurance, and Homeowners Insurance. There are other types of insurance, too, like Pet Insurance and Long-Term Care Insurance.

To be prepared for any health emergency or accident, it's advisable to have insurance to help cover the cost of any types of expenses that may come up. For example, our car got a big chip in the windshield, which ended up making big cracks. The windshield had to be replaced. Our insurance deductible was $500. The windshield cost $1,300. Thank goodness we had that insurance. Otherwise, we would have been another $800 out of pocket. Insurance premiums may seem like a waste of money at the time but can give you peace of mind.

Older adults and their P.O.A. must carefully read life-insurance policies because there may be an upper age limit that will invalidate the policy. For instance, there are policies that won't pay for anyone older than eighty-five. Also, there are several older people and deceased individuals with unclaimed funds accounts in the state's unclaimed funds inventory. Mary L. Beal of MLBeal Consulting, from Georgia, shared a story with me about her late mother's estate. The insurance company her mom had been dealing with had gone out of business years before her death. The cash surrender value was sent to the State of Georgia Department of Revenue Unclaimed Funds Office. Mary was able to get $500 before her mom passed away at age 101 and seven months in 2011. It took about six weeks, and it didn't cost her mom anything to do it. Mary was aware of the process, as it is a service she provides through her consulting business. She says it can be costly and time-consuming for heirs to collect these funds that may rightfully belong to them, according to the state's inheritance laws.

Sitting down with a trusted financial advisor or banker can help you review your current situation and long-term goals. Choose an advisor certified in the field and who is not employed by a firm that sells securities. Otherwise, their focus will be on selling you mutual funds or annuities that will make them a large commission but likely leave you with some undesirable investments. Saving money while at the same time paying off debt sounds far-fetched, but it can be done as long as you are mindful of your spending habits.

Budgets can help you stay on track and meet your overall goals. Putting money into investments can also help you save your money and help it grow. Buying stocks in the latest and greatest technology or other up-and-coming companies can also be a way to grow your money. It can be a bit of a gamble, but if done right, you can do very well. If you have any extra cash or inheritance, you may want to invest in property.

Poverty is a real and serious issue. Not having enough money for shelter, food, clean water, and clothing can affect one's health and well-being. Homelessness is also another societal issue that is related to financial insecurity. Some people are at risk of eviction if they can't afford to pay rent.

Keep an eye out for money "leakage." This happens when you are paying for services on a monthly basis that you aren't using or forget about. This includes gym memberships, T.V. or streaming-service subscriptions, landline telephone, or security monitoring services. Sometimes it takes some detective work to find out where the leak is!

If you are tight on money or watching your spending, try to find free or low-cost things to do. Here are some examples:

1. Go for a walk, pick wildflowers, and put them in a vase.

2. Participate in geocaching (worldwide outdoor treasure hunting using a Global Positioning System) to find containers holding items called geocaches or caches.

3. Go to the library.

4. Barter (equal and equitable exchange of goods or services) with your friends and those you trust.

5. Exercise at home, so you don't have to pay for a gym membership.

6. To save money on gas, walk or cycle.

7. Purchase your clothing at the thrift shops.

8. Watch the flyers for sales on groceries and other essentials.

9. Buy the no-name generic brand whenever you can.

10. Be more mindful of your spending habits.

11. Turn it into a game by stretching your dollar into two by being mindful. Challenge yourself to see how far you can stretch your dollar.

12. Try to "do-it-yourself" and be resourceful.

13. Buy yourself some hair clippers or barter with someone to cut your hair.

14. Host dinner and a movie, with a friend. Consider making a home-cooked meal and watching a movie on DVD in your living room.

To save some cash, my mom washes her car when it's raining. Then she vacuums it out by herself when the sun comes out. You can journal your spending habits if you want to see where your money is going and where you can cut back (just like a diet, but with money, instead.)

If you require programs or services that seem to be out of your reach financially, you can always ask if there are low-cost options such as free, sliding scale, subsidies, or grants. Some professionals offer "pro bono" work, provided for free or at a lower cost. You could also agree to try out a new service or product in return for an honest review on websites such as Amazon or Google.

Another tip is to never loan money to a person who has obvious problems (such as gambling addiction) who promises to pay you back with monthly interest. My grandmother had a hairdresser, Lisa, who asked to borrow $50,000 CAD to "go towards her business." She told my grandmother, in tears, that she was in debt and would "lose it all" if she didn't come up with the cash. My kind, generous, and trusting grandmother agreed to lend her the money, and she did not discuss it with her adult children (my mom and uncle).

One day, the hairdresser came by with the real estate agent, and they took my grandmother out. They took her to the bank, and the hairdresser's son co-signed the loan. My grandmother was high and excited. She felt empowered that she was able to help someone.

About two years later, my grandmother admitted that she had lent Lisa money, and the payments weren't coming in. She was factual and angry. My mom (her daughter) said, "We should report this to the police!" She agreed to have the police involved. The police attended and documented what happened. The police went after Lisa, and the bank got involved. The courts ordered Lisa to pay the $50,000 back with interest. She couldn't, so her son, who co-signed, had to. They came up with only about $39,000 altogether.

Later we found out Lisa had a gambling problem and was thousands in debt. It came to light the real estate agent and the hairdresser were working together on scamming my grandmother of thousands of dollars. We later learned the real estate agent had overcharged my grandmother $15,000 on each house she sold to her over the years.

If you are a parent or grandparent, you may want to safeguard your bank account from being taken advantage of by your children. What can start as a small amount, a "lending" situation, can eventually turn into having your bank account cleaned out. I heard about a granddaughter wiping out her grandfather's bank account, and he did not want to press charges against her. Families can be complicated. It's always important to keep in mind whom you are giving your money to and why. Having a written contract when lending money to someone is also a good idea.

Gifting your money (or possessions) is also an option, but you have to be aware of the consequences. "Giving" one child or grandchild money, a car, or another item of value can lead to family conflict. If one child hears about another getting a gift of money, she or he may consider that as unfair. This simple act can cause repercussions and bad feelings you may never have considered. If possible, it's best to gift equally, so no one gets upset.

Always be on your guard in terms of making a down payment for goods or services. Learn from me. We needed new windows for our house, so I did what I thought was the best way to find the best deal and the most trusted company. I asked for referrals from my friends, and I also looked up reputable companies on the internet.

My boss at the time suggested a company I will call A.B.C. Windows. She had them do her windows and was happy with the cost and service. I included A.B.C. Windows in my search for three quotes. They came out with flying colours, plus, my boss had referred and recommended them.

I called them up, and the owner came by and took measurements. He told us it would cost $13,000. When it came time to give the down payment, we decided to provide him with 50%—$6,000. We wrote a cheque. A few weeks later, we hadn't heard anything, so my husband called the company. There was no answer.

It turns out we had been duped. The company had gone under, and although we went to court, we didn't have a leg to stand on because the company was in receivership, and they had no assets left. There went our nice winter vacation, "out the window," so to speak. We were very upset.

The advice I would have moving forward is to inquire if you can secure the goods or services without a down payment. And if you need to provide a down payment to get the process moving, put down the bare minimum, and use a credit card. Credit-card companies will get you your money back if you do not receive the services or goods you had paid for. Your cash is as good as gone if something goes wrong.

In some states in the U.S.A., I've heard that the "legal" down payment to a contractor is 10% of the job, or $1,000—whichever is less (e.g., California). Others can request a deposit of one-third of the contract price (e.g., Maryland). Fifty percent is excessive. Check out what the law is in your jurisdiction. And don't forget to get your quote in writing (or email).

Speaking of credit cards, some come with excellent insurance features. For example, they may come with theft or loss insurance. We bought my son some eyeglasses on our credit card, and soon after, he broke them. We were able to put forward a damage claim through our credit card company, and we got the glasses replaced for no charge! One of our credit cards comes with bonus features such as Travel Emergency Medical Insurance and Car Rental Collision/Loss Damage Waiver Insurance. When looking for the best credit card, check into the additional features, interest rate, and annual fee.

Depending on your comfort level with speaking of matters related to your death, you may want to consider pre-planning your funeral. This way, when the time comes, your loved ones won't have to worry about finding the funds or deciding what to do at a very difficult time. Financial preparedness and planning ahead can help the situation. The book *I'm Dead, Now What? Important Information about My Belongings, Business Affairs, and Wishes* helps you gather all of the vital information needed for peace of mind. I am sure there are others like it. Just make sure you keep the information updated and your closest relatives know how to access this invaluable planner. Your Power of Attorney and Executor of your will should both know how to access it.

If you happen to have several assets, investments, and other financial dealings, it would be a good idea to keep them all in one place. I keep an electronic copy of all my financial and related matters on my computer. It's stored away on a password-protected site (such as Google Docs). I am a person who thinks, "What if I got hit by a truck tomorrow and died? How would my partner know the details of our financial situation?" So, he knows I take care of organizing our finances and keep all the information in one safe place. I also make sure he knows where it is, should he need to access it.

Sitting down with your financial advisor, bank, or credit-union representative can help you decide how to optimize your financial wellness. Getting a safe-deposit box can also help you safeguard any of your legal documents, precious family heirlooms, or other valuables. If you choose to go with a home safe, make sure it can withstand a house fire (ask a firefighter first). A home alarm system and/or security camera can also help protect you, your home, family, pets, and valuables. If you are fortunate enough to have savings or other investments and assets, protecting them for future generations and those whom you pass them along to can help keep you feeling confident about what you will leave behind as part of your legacy.

Financial-Wellness Self-Assessment

On a scale of 1 to 4, 1 being very dissatisfied, 4 being very satisfied, where are you at in terms of satisfaction with your financial situation?

Circle one:

1 = Very dissatisfied. Horrible. Nonexistent.
2 = Dissatisfied. Not that great.
3 = Satisfied. It's okay.
4 = Very satisfied. Very content. Happy.

Financial-Wellness Reflection

If you score on the bottom half of the scale, what can you do, moving forward, to improve your Financial-Wellness score? And when do you want to start making changes? How important is this to you? If you are scoring in the top half of the scale, what can you do to move toward a "four"?

Affirmations

- I am financially secure.
- I am preparing for my future.
- I learn all I can about financial issues.
- I am paying off my debt.
- I save for what I want.

- I need what I have and have what I need.
- I know lots of things I can do that don't cost money.

Things to Try

- Set up a meeting with a trusted financial advisor to go over your long-term financial goals.
- Commit to spending less and saving more.
- Be mindful of the "leakage" and make "repairs" regularly.
- Review all of your spending habits, and see where you can cut back.
- Plan for your retirement.
- Save for something special.
- If you want a credit card, choose one that has no annual fee and gives you money back.

Reference

Jebb, A. T., Diener, E., Oishi, S., and Tay, L. (2018). "Happiness Income Satiation, and Turning Points Around the World." *Nature Human Behaviour*, 2(1): 33-38.

Chapter 12

Occupational Wellness

Finding and creating your life's work, even if it is entirely different from what you have done most of your life, will bring you more happiness and health than any other action you can take. If your primary responsibility in life is being true to yourself, that can only be accomplished by carrying out what you are called to do—your unique and special vocation.... Your life's work involves doing what you love and loving what you do.

— Dennis Kimbro

I f you check into any of the university websites, you will most likely find a form of a "wellness wheel" that helps students balance their lives in the areas of mind, body, and soul. University students can get caught up in the stress of studying and the pressure of due dates for papers and exams, so they benefit from being reminded that, to have a good sense of overall wellness, it's a good idea to aim for balance in all areas of life. We rarely see the comprehensive wellness wheel that includes occupational—"life's work"—as the student has yet to discover and follow their dreams of a career.

Occupational Wellness, or life's work, is a vital aspect of our total wellness. Our life's work helps give us purpose, meaning, fulfilment, and money to pay the bills. It's how we "occupy" the bulk of our time. If we are lucky, and with good planning, we can get all of these needs met (even in retirement).

After we get out of school and find a significant other (not necessarily in that order!), we may end up in the role of housewife, stay-at-home mom, or working outside the home. Or one may experience a combination of all of that. I worked part-time at the beginning of my career, and I was also a part-time stay-at-home mom when the kids were little.

For those of us in our later years, we have already had a job or career, possibly many jobs and careers, so it's important for us to take a closer look at where we are at with our "job" or "vocation." Life's work for us older folks could mean many things, and it changes over the lifespan.

Life's Work

- ♦ Job
- ♦ Vocation
- ♦ Calling
- ♦ Career
- ♦ Profession
- ♦ Trade
- ♦ Volunteerism
- ♦ Retirement
- ♦ Learning
- ♦ Teaching
- ♦ Roles
- ♦ Purpose
- ♦ Caregiving

The need to work and be employed is thoroughly ingrained in North America's culture and customs. For those who can't work, we have families or other social systems to help people get their basic needs met. Having a vocation or a calling to do some kind of work, either paid or unpaid, gives us a sense of purpose and helps put food on our table and a song in our hearts.

When we are young, it's expected that we find a job. Going to school—finishing high school, for example—is part of a bigger plan to help us get the life skills we need to read, write, do math, and attain other basic life skills (such as sex education!). This prepares us to go forth into the world and be productive members of society. For some of us, seeking post-secondary education such as college, university, or learning trades is something we work hard toward.

Dreams of becoming a doctor or a teacher can be realized by putting in some focused study and commitment. Depending on how your parents raised you, you may or may not have been encouraged to seek higher education. You may have been encouraged toward—or were simply more interested in—playing sports. Maybe the arts were more your thing. Our parents' job is to give us the support and skills we need to "launch" and move on with our lives. Finding a job or a place in our world sometimes takes time and a few tries before we succeed.

We may go through a few jobs in our lifetime. Continuing education and professional development can help us reach our goals if we want to change careers or move up in our current position. Some jobs may be rewarding; some may be stressful; some may be just okay. The good thing about jobs is, we have a choice. If you are in a position you don't like, you can always consider changing it.

I had a job in home care for nine years before realizing it was not the right fit for me. I was burning out. Stress, governmental red tape, and bureaucracy limited my ability to help others in a practical, meaningful way. I set out to find a new job, as I wanted out—badly. I ended up becoming burnt out, and I had to take a stress leave. It was a devastating time in my life. I felt like a complete failure, and I felt ashamed that I couldn't "take the heat." I wondered what was wrong with me. After I decided, in my mind, that I was going to quit that job on a specific date whether I had another job to go to or not, I luckily found another job—one year later—that was a better fit for me. It suited my lifestyle, income needs, interests, and expertise. My stress was lifted, and I felt much better. I underwent what I would call a "Career Shift."

We all have roles and jobs in our own homes. If you live alone, all the responsibilities will fall onto you. If you live with someone else, those roles may be divided or shared. For example, my husband takes out the garbage on Sundays, and I do the laundry on the weekends. In some homes, cooking and cleaning are shared, and one person handles the finances. One or the other may be more inclined to do the yard work, and others may do the grocery shopping. When there are pets and children, you may give an older child the job of feeding or walking the pet. Kids can help unload the dishwasher or sweep the floor. No matter what roles or jobs you have around your household, these are essential life skills you have, and these jobs matter!

You can also find meaning and fulfillment in volunteer work. There are many opportunities for those who want to donate their time or skills without pay to benefit others. Being of service to others can make us feel happy. I have a good friend who is a retired accountant and volunteers on a large healthcare facility board. Formal volunteer programs can provide you with added supervision and support. Being part of a larger group of volunteers can also enrich your life as it offers opportunities to connect with others who are like-minded. Volunteer recognition is also a good feeling!

I have volunteered for many organizations. When I was in university, one of my first volunteer experiences was with the "Big Sisters Association." I was matched up with a young girl who needed a "big sister" in her life. It was a great program (and it looked good on my resume). I have been involved with many other volunteer programs over the years, and they have all been rewarding.

Lifelong learning is strongly encouraged for brain health and personal development. Ask any teacher. Learning to play the piano and practicing regularly is a skill that you will have all your life, and no one can take it away from you. Taking a course on world religions can enrich your understanding of others' views. Deciding to teach a class or a skill to others is also an excellent way to learn something. Writing a book like this has helped me develop my teaching skills while sharing in the written word what I have learned over the years. Any time we learn, teach, or are open to hearing about new things, we are flexing our brain—and our brain needs flexing no matter how old we are!

Attitudes towards retirement are changing. The dream of "Freedom 55" is a reality for many. Many people who speak of retiring say it with a sparkle in their eye and a smile on their face. Some retire at the "normal" age of 65. Others are choosing to work past the age of 65. I once told a friend that I wished that it was me retiring, and she replied, "But I don't think you'd want to be this age." I sensed the sadness in her voice. She is planning on working on a casual basis after her mandatory six-week retirement. A widely used term for this is "double-dipping," and it's perfectly legal. People can receive their Canada Pension Plan and employer pension benefit and also earn additional income. They can choose to work as much or as little as they want.

The experience and expertise of people who have worked in a given field is invaluable, and some skill sets are very desirable. Many of us will be working for 25 to 30 years or even more. It's a good idea to speak with a banker or financial advisor before retiring to see if you can afford it. If there is a significant other in your life, make sure you discuss your plans him or her as well. If we have planned right, we can retire from our "regular" job and feel the freedom of doing whatever we want.

There are many reasons why people retire. Some like to wait until they are 65 because that's just what people do. Others have health problems, so they retire earlier. When both of my parents were in their mid-70s and still working, I asked them, "When do you plan on retiring?" My dad said, "When my legs give out." My mom said, "I will work for as long as I am physically able." Some want to (or need to) stay home to look after ailing relatives or provide childcare to grandchildren. Some people want an "encore career." If done right, retirement can provide you with a pension and the ability to do a different job (if your health allows). Maybe you want to start your own business or consulting firm. Perhaps you want to get out of a stressful healthcare career as a nurse and move into a less-stressful job or volunteer position such as being a guide at the local museum.

No matter what you end up doing with the bulk of your time, I suggest that you seek out something meaningful and rewarding. Going back to school full-time to get that degree you always wanted isn't too far-fetched. Switching careers or retiring with a plan (or no plan for some!) are other options. If your choice is to stay home and watch TV, that's okay, too! However, if you love the work you are doing now, and the routine is right for you, I hope you can continue doing it as long as you want!

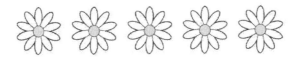

Occupational-Wellness Self-Assessment

On a scale of 1 to 4, 1 being very dissatisfied, 4 being very satisfied, where are you at in terms of satisfaction with your occupational wellness?

Circle one:

1 = Very dissatisfied. Horrible. Nonexistent.
2 = Dissatisfied. Not that great.
3 = Satisfied. It's okay.
4 = Very satisfied. Very content. Happy.

Occupational-Wellness Reflection

If you score on the bottom half of the scale, what can you do, moving forward, to improve your Occupational-Wellness score? And when do you want to start making changes? How important is this to you? If you are scoring in the top half of the scale, what can you do to move toward a "four"?

Affirmations

- I have a great job.
- I am looking for a rewarding job.
- My life's work is meaningful.
- I find purpose in my career.
- I am retired and loving it.
- I like how I spend the bulk of my time.
- I am retiring with a plan.
- I am going to work as long as I can.
- I have roles in my home, and it's working for me.

Things to Try

- Find a volunteer job that fits in with your life.
- Determine whether you like your job or not, and if you don't, change either your job or your attitude.
- Sign up for a course to help you learn a new skill.
- Think about how long you want to stay in your current job, and consider what you will do upon retirement.
- Dust off and update your résumé.
- Write or draw what your "dream job" would be.
- Talk to others who are retired, and ask them how they like it.

Chapter 13

How to Complete a Self-Assessment

How Do You Score on the Ten Dimensions of Wellness?

Supplies needed:

•   Blank paper or journal, pen or pencil

The *Flower of Wellness* Method is a self-assessment for women at midlife and beyond. You will need to have a good understanding of 10 dimensions of wellness: Physical, Emotional, Brain, Social, Sexual, Spiritual, Environmental, Recreational, Financial, and Occupational. Keep in mind no one dimension is more important than another. They all influence, overlap, and interface with each other. They are interconnected. You may place more emphasis on one or two dimensions than the others in your life, and that's okay!

Strive for satisfaction in *all* areas, based on your subjective and personalized self-assessment.

Note: If you find another dimension that is more important to you not listed here, please feel free to add it to your flower, or substitute it for another as you see necessary. It's your life.

After reading through each chapter listed above, you will have a good understanding of the essence of each dimension. Each dimension represents a petal on the *Flower of Wellness*. Reflect on your life, and consider how satisfied you are in each area. Choose your score from 1 to 4, with 1 being least satisfied and 4 being most satisfied. Jot down your answers here, or if you prefer, write down your answers on a piece of paper or in your journal.

1 = Very dissatisfied. Horrible. Nonexistent.
2 = Dissatisfied. Not that great.
3 = Satisfied. It's okay.
4 = Very satisfied. Very content. Happy.

_____ Physical
_____ Emotional
_____ Brain
_____ Social
_____ Sexual
_____ Spiritual
_____ Environmental
_____ Recreational
_____ Financial
_____ Occupational

There are two ways to analyze this information.

Method 1: *Flower of Wellness* Score Analysis

You can look at the numbers above and complete a *Flower of Wellness* score analysis. Threes and fours mean you are satisfied. Ones and twos, not satisfied. Hopefully, you will have a few threes and fours. These are areas you are thriving and doing well in. You will likely also notice there are areas for improvement. These are the areas you may want to focus on. Keep in mind, even if you scored a 3 or 4, there may still be room for growth and improvement.

Go back to the corresponding chapter for each dimension you are least satisfied with. At the end of each chapter is a list of *Affirmations* and *Things to Try*. There are other questions for you to think about as well. You may come up with some of your own ideas, too.

In your journal, list a few things you would like to work on—short-term and long-term goals—highlighting one thing you could easily accomplish. When you have achieved your first goal, add this information to your journal. Go back and work on another. Add to your list as you go.

Repeat this process at least once yearly or after a major life event. You will see your flower bloom and mature as you work towards reaching total well-being.

Method 2: *Flower of Wellness* Diagram

The second method of analyzing your results will give you more of a visual image—the *Flower of Wellness* diagram. This will take a little more creativity. You will be drawing your *Flower of Wellness*. It's a simple daisy, with 10 petals. Each petal represents a dimension as listed above. The length of the petal indicates how satisfied you are with each of the areas. On the next page is a fully mature *Flower of Wellness*.

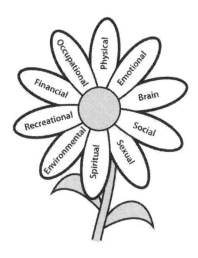

Flower of Wellness

A mature, flourishing daisy would have petals that are all the same length. One that is in the development-and-growth stage will have petals that are not yet full grown. The petals on your flower will help you see where there is room to grow.

Using your numerical answers to each of the dimensions as noted above, each rating will determine the size of the corresponding petal. There are four petal lengths. Sizes range from "small" to "extra-large."

SEVEN STEPS OF THE *FLOWER OF WELLNESS* METHOD SELF-ASSESSMENT

Step 1. Go back to each chapter, and review your answers, especially the one that asks, on a scale of 1 to 4, where are you at in terms of your satisfaction with all 10 dimensions.

1 = Very dissatisfied. Horrible. Nonexistent.
2 = Dissatisfied. Not that great.
3 = Satisfied. It's okay.
4 = Very satisfied. Very content. Happy.

Jot down the rating for each dimension (as noted earlier). Remember, there are no right or wrong answers. This is very personal and subjective. Only you know if there is room (or need) for improvement or not.

Step 2. You will be drawing a daisy, based on your answers to each of the questions. Give yourself lots of room on your page, and start with a small circle representing the centre of the daisy. This is you. You are the glue that holds everything together and where all the dimensions intersect.

Step 3. Add the 10 petals based on your self-assessment rating of each dimension (as noted above). Label each petal with the dimension it represents, in no specific order. Each rating will determine the size of the petal.

> 1 = Very Dissatisfied/Petal is 1/4 length (small)
> 2 = Dissatisfied/Petal is 1/2 length (medium)
> 3 = Satisfied/Petal is 3/4 length (large)
> 4 = Very Satisfied/Petal is full length (extra-large)

Step 4. After completing your flower diagram, take a moment to reflect and decide where there is room to grow. The smaller petals will stand out as immature and needing further development. Pick a dimension that you consider a priority, and go back to that chapter for ideas if needed. At the end of each chapter are lists of *Affirmations* and *Things to Try*. There are other questions for you to think about as well. You may want to look at a couple of areas and decide what will be most beneficial. You may come up with some of your own ideas, too.

Step 5. Pledge to yourself that you will commit to improving something that will help move you towards a sense of total well-being. Pick one dimension to work on. List a few things you would like to do—short-term and long-term goals—highlighting one thing you could easily accomplish. Write your goals in your journal or on a piece of paper. You don't have to start with anything too big or complicated. Small and easy successes, which I call "low-hanging fruit," can strengthen your self-improvement muscles and self-confidence. Celebrate each step. When you have achieved your first goal, check it off in your journal. Go back and work on another. Add to your list as you go.

Step 6. When ready, tackle another issue or dimension that seems more meaningful to you. It may take a little more work, but it will help get you to a sense of total well-being. Repeat this process until you feel you are more satisfied and happier. Celebrate your accomplishments, no matter how big or small.

Step 7. When you feel you have addressed all the dimensions that needed some attention, congratulate yourself on a job well done! You are *flourishing, not fading.*

Example: *Flower of Wellness* Diagram for Jane

Jane is 57 and single. She started by drawing a small circle in the middle of her paper. Then she went back and looked at the score for each dimension (order doesn't matter). Jane just retired, and she feels great about it, so she scores a 4 (very satisfied) for Occupational and Emotional Wellness. Both of these petals are extra-large, and she labeled them. For Social Wellness, Jane scored a 3, which means she is satisfied in that area, and that petal is almost mature. She is also very satisfied (a score of 4) in other dimensions, such as Financial and Spiritual, but she feels that Brain and Physical need some work (dissatisfied, with a score of 2). The Environmental dimension is at a three. She is not happy with her Sexual Wellness and gave that a two. Since she is retired, she will be working on Recreational Wellness, which she gives a score of three. Jane's flower looks like it needs a little more time to fully develop and flourish. On the next page is Jane's diagram.

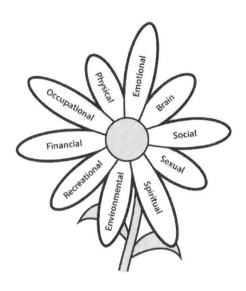

Jane's *Flower of Wellness*

This provides a visual of where there is room for improvement. Perhaps Jane could do a little more in the Social Wellness area and join a women's group. She could increase her satisfaction with Physical Wellness by going for a brisk 20-minute walk daily and cutting back on sweets. Learning about and purchasing a composter could help improve her Environmental Wellness. Jane could review each relevant chapter for ideas for how she could improve her overall well-being.

Repeat Regularly

Repeat the *Flower of Wellness* self-assessment process regularly, at least once a year. If you experience a significant lifestyle change, such as a divorce, retirement, or disability, you may want to revisit this self-assessment sooner than the one-year mark. It can help you stay balanced and flourishing, even through difficult times.

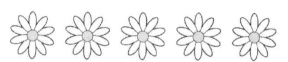

Chapter 14

Conclusion: A Better Plan for Aging Well

Self-awareness and self-assessment are two main factors in a successful journey of self-improvement. Learning about the interconnected dimensions of wellness and applying what you have learned to your situation can help you make some positive changes in your life.

We can't expect changes to happen quickly, because in most cases, the challenges or dissatisfactions didn't develop overnight. It has most likely taken years to get to this stage, so be gentle with yourself. Self-compassion and self-care are of the utmost importance when working on personal development. Keep in mind that one small change can mean a considerable improvement in your overall health and wellness.

Review and revisit the 10 dimensions of wellness regularly, at least once yearly. Keep yourself engaged and active, living your best life.

Then, when and if you are ready, check out the Appendix titled "Being Prepared," and make some plans for your future.

Today is the first day of the rest of your life. Commit to making the rest of your life the best of your life.

If you need more time and would like to read some more, please check out the Recommended Reading list and the Online Resources.

Appendix

Being Prepared—
Let's get serious

Old age ain't no place for sissies.

— Bette Davis (1908-1989)

Getting our "ducks in a row" is a popular catchphrase that suits this chapter. As we get older, there are things we can do to prepare in case of disease, infirmity, or death. Getting our affairs in order—doing those things that we tend to put off because perhaps they make us "uncomfortable"—can help us get ready for whatever the next step may be. Having these difficult, uncomfortable conversations with our loved ones can prevent frustration and stress when the time comes. These conversations, decisions, and actionable tasks can be done for ourselves, as well as for our loved ones. "Senior orphans"—those without children, a spouse, or significant other—will have additional challenges. I will present some topic areas that are important for us to consider at midlife and beyond and for our older loved ones, such as our parents. (This chapter may also be appropriate for your parents or older loved ones to read.)

Home Safety

Everyone needs a roof over their head and a place to call home. At some point, we may need to downsize and move to an apartment or a smaller home. Housing for seniors can offer amenities that improve safety and security. Depending on your income, you may have more freedom in your choices, or you may need to consider rent-geared-to-income or subsidized offerings. Moving in with someone or having someone move in with you (e.g., a live-in caregiver) might be your best option.

At some point, there may be safety issues with living at home alone, but you may have decided that moving somewhere else is not desirable. Some things can be done to improve independent living. Getting a personal alarm to wear on your wrist or a pendant can give you peace of mind if you have a bad fall or other emergency. Giving a house key to a trusted family member or friend can help them get in if need be. Hiding a key outside the home under a mat, rock, or planter also works for some people. Getting an outdoor combination lockbox for a house key is a secure option. The only thing a person needs is a code to gain access to the house key. House alarms can also improve security. Deadbolts offer added protection.

Talking to an older loved one about your concerns about them living on their own can be difficult. Perhaps you're afraid they'll fall down the stairs. Can the washer and dryer be brought up to the main level? Are you concerned they may leave the stove on and burn something? Consider getting them meal delivery, or have Home Care helpers come in to reheat their meals. The fuse for the stove can be removed, or it can be unplugged if it gets to be a real concern.

Accessing community resources and home care services can be a bit difficult, and navigating the system can be overwhelming. Your local senior services organization, healthcare provider, or a simple Google search can help you find local resources suited to your situation.

I have prepared a list of risks for those who live independently at home. If any of these risks are present, it may be time to either problem-solve (such as adding additional resources) or have the person move to a more supportive environment such as enhanced assisted living, supportive housing, or a long-term care residence.

Driving Cessation

Driving is a privilege. Many older people start to lose their cognitive abilities to operate a motor vehicle safely. Their decision-making or navigational skills may be impaired. They may get lost or get into accidents. Perhaps their vision is declining. Having a conversation with a loved one about "retiring from driving" can be difficult, especially when the person has been driving for 60 years! I have had to alert family doctors about my concerns, so sometimes it's the family doctor who either pulls the license or refers the person for driver's testing.

If you are considering retiring from driving, it's important to establish an alternate transportation plan. Whether it's taking taxis, having a friend or family member do the driving, or hiring a driver, having a reliable alternative for how you will get around is imperative. Being told you can't drive anymore can feel like the worst thing in the world; not having an alternative will make it even worse. I have also seen people appeal the decision and fight to get their license back. This usually does not end well.

For those with a diagnosis of dementia, you may need to hide their keys or disable their car (e.g., disconnect the wires that go to the battery, remove the battery, or put a steering-wheel club on it). One family arrived at a creative solution by telling their 90-year-old father that the "car is in the shop." It was there for a long time—long enough for him to get used to safe and alternative ways to get around. The conversation about driving cessation needs to take place before a person becomes unsafe behind the wheel.

Moving to a Nursing Home

Most people detest the idea of moving to a "nursing home." Aging in place is what most of us prefer and want for ourselves and our loved ones. A few families I have worked with over the years have told me their parent asked them to promise they will "never put me in a home." I would advise you never to ask your children to promise you that. A nursing home is a last resort for anyone, and there are only a very few people who have ever *wanted* to go to one. In fact, only about 4.5% of the entire population of older adults live in nursing homes. Considering this fact, the chances of going to one are very slim.

The 24-hour nursing care residences I have worked in are often filled to capacity, and a majority of the people are very old and physically and mentally unwell. Many of the people there have had a stroke or have severe arthritis or other kinds of physical challenges. These are people who need constant supervision and assistance with many of the activities of daily living, such as getting dressed/undressed, bathing, taking medicine, getting meals/eating, etc. A majority of them have some form of dementia, such as Alzheimer's disease. Sometimes they wander in and out of other residents' rooms, and they may get into altercations with other residents or staff (due to their inability to accurately interpret their situation and their environment.)

Having a conversation with your loved ones about your wishes and their wishes is uncomfortable, but it will help save your family grief and stress when and if the time comes for a decision to be made about housing. I will never tell my family, "Don't ever put me in a home." Instead, I will give them the authority to do what they think is in my best interest. I won't make them struggle and burn out because I made them promise not to place me in a nursing or personal care home. It can cost a lot of money to have someone cared for 24/7 in their residence. It also causes stress and worries for those responsible for organizing the care and troubleshooting as needed. It's truly a 24/7 job.

Moving someone to a long-term care environment can be stressful and expensive, but sometimes the choice has to be made for the mental health and well-being of those involved. Touring homes ahead of time can help you make a wise and sound decision. Some homes have better reputations than others for staffing, amenities, food, and services.

As an aside, to make a stay at a home more pleasant, you may want to make photo albums of favourite people and places, generally referred to as a "Memory Box." Label the pictures so that, when it comes time to reminisce—especially if the person's memory skills are waning—it will be easier to retrieve those names and memories. Include in your Memory Box a list of favourite music, programs/movies, and other trinkets or items that brought joy. These favourites can come in handy down the road.

I was absolutely stunned when I saw a beautiful quilt that was made out of ties. A man had kept more than 100 ties in his closet, and after he passed, his daughter found them. She had his ties made into a quilt, and now it sits in her mom's living room. Family heirlooms such as favourite tops, blankets, small wooden tables, photographs, paintings, and the like can help bring back fond memories. Framing certificates received on special occasions, such as 50th wedding anniversaries or celebrating 20 years of service with a company, are also great conversation starters. Family portraits are always a hit, too!

A list of your bank accounts, social-media accounts, investments (and associated passwords) should be kept in a safe place. You may have a safe deposit box with an extra key that you want to share with a trusted individual (in case you are unable to act on your own behalf). I use a philosophy called, "What if I was hit by a truck tomorrow?" I want to make sure my loved ones know where all the important papers and passwords are kept in case something happens to me. No one knows when or how their time will come, so keeping this in mind, while uncomfortable, is a loving and kind gesture to those who would be left behind.

Power of Attorney

One of the most critical documents I strongly recommend is a Power of Attorney (P.O.A.). Depending on where you live, this could be for your financial and estate matters only, or it could be for your personal care as well. Banks also give P.O.A. for specific financial accounts and affairs.

In Manitoba, we have a Power of Attorney for estate and financial affairs. This is a legal document that requires a lawyer's signature.

If you ever become unable to make your own decisions, the person to whom you have assigned P.O.A. will be able to act on your behalf. The P.O.A. should be "enduring" or "durable," which means if you have a stroke, get into a bad accident, slip into a coma, or become incapacitated due to mental illness or dementia, the P.O.A. you have entrusted will be able to use her or his authority without a doctor's note.

If the P.O.A. is "springing" (which I do not recommend), then the P.O.A. will need two doctors' opinions indicating you are no longer able to manage your affairs. That can put the family member (or whoever you appoint as P.O.A.) in a difficult spot. Finding two doctors can take time, which causes more problems, especially when trying to sell property or real estate.

When appointing a P.O.A., you can pick one person (e.g., your spouse) as primary and another as an alternate. If the first person is not available or capable of acting on your behalf, the authority will go to the second person. If you have two people (e.g., a daughter and a son) appointed as your P.O.A., they can be listed as an "or" or an "and," which means "jointly." When you speak to your lawyer about getting this done, make sure you understand the implications of the decisions you make regarding "alternate," "or," "jointly," and "enduring." There are other options to consider, such as whether this person can decide where you live. The P.O.A. can delegate someone else to carry out their responsibilities. The other family members can ask the P.O.A. for an accounting of their loved one's banking and estate matters.

Power of Attorney for personal care is also known as a Medical P.O.A., Advance Health Care Directive, or Living Will. There are two parts. Your medical-treatment wishes will be spelled out, and you will assign someone on your behalf to act as your "Healthcare Proxy." Your P.O.A. for healthcare decisions will be the person who speaks on your behalf, should you be unable to make sound and rational decisions about your healthcare. For more information on Advance Care Planning, check out the website "Speak Up Canada" (advancecareplanning.ca).

You may have already made it clear that you want "no heroic measures" if you cannot breathe on your own (e.g., no intubation or life support). A Living Will comes into effect when you cannot express yourself verbally, physically, or in writing. You may also be deemed incompetent if you have dementia or an acute illness rendering you incapacitated. Having a conversation with your loved ones about your medical-care wishes will help make the process easier if or when the time ever comes. Perhaps you want to have medicine for an easily treated problem like a bladder infection. However, you may not want invasive biopsies, surgeries, or radiation should you experience a recurrence of cancer.

Some people do not have legal P.O.A. documents or Advance Health Care Directives when they become incapacitated. In that case, they will require a legal guardian or substitute decision-maker to be appointed by a judge to manage their affairs and person. A family member can apply for this role and can appeal to the courts.

In Manitoba, we have a provincial government organization called the Public Guardian and Trustee of Manitoba, which employs officers who will help manage a person's affairs. The terminology is different depending on where you live, so the legally appointed person or entity could be referred to as a "conservator" or some other related term. Consulting a doctor, lawyer, or geriatric social worker are options if you are unsure who to turn to.

A simple and easy step to making things smoother at the end of life is adding a trusted family member as a joint account or titleholder. For example, if you have a checking account in your name only, and something happens to you, your family would not have easy access to your money. Making an appointment at the bank and putting your trusted son's or daughter's name on the account (joint bank account) makes it much easier for them to access this money if needed. You can also put their name on the house title or any other assets you have. Ensuring you have the correct benefactors listed on insurance policies will also aid in a smoother, less-stressful experience. A financial advisor or accountant can help make sure all of these things are taken care of.

End-of-life issues are difficult to talk about, but if you should ever find yourself or a loved one in this situation, it makes it a lot easier to deal with if you have had those conversations. I often think if I had late-stage dementia and I no longer wanted to eat, I would not want to be tube-fed or force-fed. I would want nature to take its course.

For a person whose death is imminent, perhaps they want to die at home. Careful planning and discussion with the healthcare team can help ensure there are palliative or hospice services available to ensure comfort and support. If the person does not want to be resuscitated, a "Do not resuscitate" order (D.N.R.) should be in place. An Advance Health Care Directive or Living Will are documents that you can complete to help make sure your wishes are followed in the event of a medical illness or emergency.

Preparing a Last Will or Trust will ensure your wishes are made known in terms of what happens to your possessions and assets when you have passed. You will appoint an executor (and an alternate) to deal with your affairs. The executor will arrange to pay your bills, distribute your possessions, liquidate what needs to be (cars, house, jewelry, etc.), deal with the bank, and help tie up any other loose ends (e.g., income tax.) The executor has a role of great responsibility, so make sure you have chosen a trusted and capable individual.

Funeral arrangements can be made ahead of time. Having a discussion with your loved ones about your wishes (cremation, burial, etc.) can help those who have to make decisions at a very sad and stressful time. Talking about what kind of service you want, or if you prefer a Celebration of Life or no service at all, can offer direction to those who will have to manage after you have passed. Having this conversation with your close relatives, such as your parents, is also a good idea. Writing down their wishes will ensure you get the details correct. It's even possible to pre-pay your funeral expenses. Some employment or government programs also include death benefits. This can go towards covering the cost of a funeral or other burial expenses. When you or a loved one dies, the funeral home should provide a list of things that need to be done.

You will want to make sure your loved ones know where your important documents are kept. For example, I keep my Will, Power of Attorney, and Advance Health Care Directive in a safe-deposit box at the bank. My family knows where this safe-deposit box is and where the key is kept.

I received a sample document of a "Procedure at Death" from Mary L. Beal, which she said I can share (see next page). This is document contains specific instructions for a person you (Trustor) name as Trustee. Each province or state will have specific regulations, so this is just an example from the state of Georgia.

Things to Do Before You Die

Have you ever thought about what you will be remembered for when you are gone? You may want to consider what kind of legacy you would like to leave. For instance, if you want to write a book, paint pictures, make music, write down some recipes—these are all things that you will be remembered by. You can even plan to save or enhance many lives by donating your tissues or organs. In the name of science, you may want to apply to donate your body for health-science education. Yes, this is something you may have to apply for! Your will could have some specific instructions to give money from your estate to one of your favourite causes or charities. You could ask your family to request donations to a particular cause instead of flowers.

My friend's mom made a special request before she died. She asked that she be cremated and her ashes buried under a tree that would feed the birds. As per her wishes, instead of a traditional burial, the family planted a beautiful Mountain Ash at their cottage. Mom's ashes were placed in the soil under the tree that produces red berries. This tree is a beautiful way to remember her.

PROCEDURE AT DEATH OF TRUSTOR

Name: _____

Birthdate: _____

Place of Birth: _____

Social Security Number: _____

Military Service Number: _____

At my death, the successor Trustee is requested to do the following:

1. Contact my attorney or other person who holds instructions in case of my death whose name is listed in the Trust and/or Will. S/he will help with the following:

   a. Proceed now with steps to take to avoid probate.
   b. Advise if there is a need to file death tax forms, either federal or state government.
   c. Assist in transferring assets to the beneficiaries of the Trust.
   d. Remove my name from jointly held assets.

2. Apply with the Social Security Office for any death or survivor benefits.
3. Call each life insurance company or agent, advising them of my death.
4. Be prepared to obtain value (or appraisal) of each asset as of the date of my death, if requested to do so by my attorney.
5. It is usually helpful to secure between three and eight certified copies of my death certificate.
6. The following special funeral instructions are requested:
7. My successor Trustee, as listed in my Trust, should be notified immediately.
8. My other miscellaneous instructions and requests are as follows:

_____

_____, Trustor   Date:_____

Share your thoughts and feelings with your family members about what you would want. This is a gift to each other. When you are ready, and the timing seems right, start by saying something like, "I've been thinking about the future. I was wondering if you would be okay with talking to me about some serious stuff." Hopefully, this kind of approach will get the discussion started. And when you are ready to put pen to paper, make sure the person's wishes are clear!

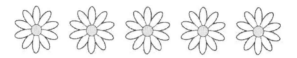

Things to Try

- Have a discussion with your family about your wishes.
- Ask your parents about their wishes.
- Prepare or update your documents (Will, Power of Attorney, Living Will, etc.)
- Put all your important documents and passwords in a safe place, and let your family know where they are kept.
- Watch some videos about how to talk to your parents about sensitive subjects (see suggestions in resources below).

Important Information Storage Systems Resources

Peter Pauper Press (2014). *I Am Dead. Now What?: Important information about my belongings, business affairs, and wishes.* (Book available on Amazon)

Greying Gracefully: Live Life Fully! "Listing Life Fully." https://gracefullygreying.com/product/listing-life-fully (48-page coil-bound book or ebook available)

Difficult-Conversation Resources

"The Conversation Project." It gives people a way to start the conversation. There is a conversation guide. Check out the "Conversation Starter Kit." https://theconversationproject.org

"Essential Conversations with Dr. Amy D'Aprix." This is a series of videos by a gerontological social worker, including "Talking to your parents about their finances" and "Assuming a parent wants to move in with you." The videos can be found on the Chartwell Retirement Residence website: https://chartwell.com/en/learn/expert-advice/essential-conversations-with-dr-amy

Other Resources

Mayo Clinic: "Living Wills and Advance Directives for Medical Reasons" is a great article explaining what living wills and advanced directives are. https://www.mayoclinic.org/healthy-lifestyle/consumer-health/in-depth/living-wills/art-20046303

Recommended Reading

Note: Some books are available in hardcover, paperback, and ebook format. Most are available on Amazon.

Applewhite, Ashton (2016). *This Chair Rocks: A manifesto against ageism.*

Bradley, Jacqueline (2005). *The Bombshell Bible: The Only Makeover Book for Style and Soul.*

Buettner, Dan (2008). *The Blue Zones: Lessons for living longer from the people who've lived the longest.*

Chittister, Joan (2010). *The Gift of Years: Growing Older Gracefully.*

Clarke, Laura Hurd (2010). *Facing Age: Women growing older in anti-aging culture.*

Cloutier, Marissa and Eve Adamson (2004). *The Mediterranean Diet.*

Fogler, Janet and Lynn Stern (2014). *Improving Your Memory: How to remember what you are starting to forget.*

Fotuhi, Majid (2003). *The Memory Cure: How to Protect Your Brain Against Memory Loss and Alzheimer's Disease.*

Goscicki, Camille (2018). *The Art of Sane Aging for Women: Embrace the journey.*

Heller, Marla (2014). *The Dash Diet Younger You: Shed 20 years—and pounds—in just 10 weeks.*

Kosik, Kenneth S, (2015). *Outsmarting Alzheimer's: What You Can Do to Reduce Your Risk.*

LaRoche, Loretta (2007). *Juicy Living, Juicy Aging: Kick up your heels . . . before you're too short to wear them.*

Lereah, David Alan (2020). *The Power of Positive Aging: Successfully coping with the inconveniences of aging.*

Mayo Clinic (2013). *Mayo Clinic on Healthy Aging: How to find happiness and vitality for a lifetime.*

Patchell-Evans, David (2002). *Living the Good Life: Your guide to health and success.*

Pfeiffer, Eric (2013). *Winning Strategies for Successful Aging* (Yale University Press Health & Wellness)

Price, Joan (2014). *The Ultimate Guide to Sex After Fifty: How to Maintain — or Regain — a Spicy, Satisfying Sex Life.*

Snowdon, David (2001). *Aging with Grace: What the nun study teaches us about leading longer, healthier, and more meaningful lives.*

Thomashauer, Regena (2002). *Mama Gena's School of Womanly Arts: Using the Power of Pleasure to Have Your Way with the World.*

Valliant, George E. (2003). *Aging Well: Surprising guideposts to a happier life from the landmark study of adult development.*

Weil, Andrew (2005). *Healthy Aging: A lifelong guide to your well-being.*

Wilder, Barbara (2005). *Embracing Your Power Woman: Coming of Age in the Second Half of Life. A course in Feminine Power.*

Winter, Cheryl Townsend (2013). *The Aging Gracefully Pathway: A toolkit for the journey.*

Online Resources

AARP is the nation's largest not-for-profit, nonpartisan organization dedicated to empowering Americans 50 and older to choose how they live as they age. aarp.org; carp.ca (CARP Canada)

Age International. ageinternational.org.uk

Help Age. HelpAge.org

International Council on Active Aging. icaa.cc

International Federation on Ageing. ifa.ngo

The National Institute on Aging. www.nia.nih.gov

Gracefully Greying: Living Life Fully! gracefullygreying.com

World Cancer Research Fund International. www.wcrf.org

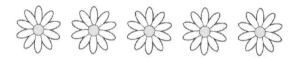

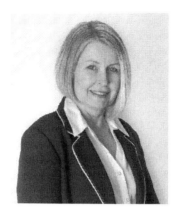

About the Author

Angela G. Gentile was born in Toronto, Ontario. She is a registered clinical social worker and obtained her B.S.W. and M.S.W. at the University of Manitoba. Her current employment is with the Winnipeg Regional Health Authority, where she is a Geriatric Mental Health Clinician.

Angela is married and has two adult children. She has written numerous articles, books, and an app for iOS. When not writing, she reads, travels, supports others online, and spends time with family and friends. Angela, who considers herself a realistic optimist, resides in Winnipeg with her husband, daughter, and two dogs.

For more information: www.AngelaGGentile.com

Other Books
by the Author

Eat Less Often, Live More: What one year of intermittent fasting taught me (2020)

Cancer Up the Wazoo: Stories, information, and hope for those affected by anal cancer (2018)

How to Edit an Anthology: Write or compile a collection that sells (2018)

Caring for a Husband with Dementia: The Ultimate Survival Guide (2015)

A Book About Burnout: One social worker's tale of survival (2015)

Mobile app co-authored with Karen Tyrell:

Dementia Caregiver Solutions (2015) (Mobile app for iOS 8 and above)

To find out how to get your copies, visit www.AngelaGGentile.com or email caretoage@gmail.com.

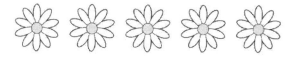

INDEX

Figures in *bold italics*.

D

dating, 86, 106, 107

death, 26, 60, 70, 75, 116, 148, 153, 175, 182-184

declutter, 128, 130, 131

delegate, 59, 180

delirium, 71, 72, 80

dementia (also see Alzheimer's disease), 18, 26, 28, 46, 52, 70-73, 76-79, 84, 85, 91, 144, 177-182, 193

denial (refusal to accept), 4

dental. *See* teeth.

dentist, 39, 47

dentures, 39

depression, 60, 61, 72, 80, 84, 85, 115

diabetes, 15, 23, 25, 26, 41, 49, 71

dietary approaches to stop hypertension (DASH), 18, 78, 187

dietician, 19, 27, 108

disability, 4, 13, 28, 147, 171

doctor visits (*also see* checkups), 24, 27, 39, 40

donations, 92, 117, 130, 145, 183

downsize, 60, 130, 175

dribbling. *See* incontinence.

driving, 38, 176-177

drug use (problematic), 4, 45, 58

dry brushing, 49

dual-energy x-ray absorptiometry (DEXA scan), 15, 30

dying, 1, 26

E

early detection, 39, 50

embrace aging, 5, 12

emergency response information kit (E.R.I.K.), 40-41

encore career (*see also* working and career shift), 161

end of life, 181

essential oils, 49, 127

estrangement, 60, 88

exfoliate, 49

eyebrows, 104, 105

eyelashes, 105

F

falls, 14, 28-32, 35, 36, 44, 176

falls prevention, 28-32

family therapy, 8

fan (the appliance), 16

fashion, 43

feet, 26, 32, 36, 37, 49, 119

5-4-3-2-1 Grounding Technique. *See* mindfulness.

flossing, 47

Flower of Wellness, 9

foot nurse, 49

forest bathing, 119, 123

forgiveness, 58, 67, 119

fracture prevention, 28-32

fragrances, 111-112, 127

frailty, 14, 15, 28, 29

funeral, 153, 182, 184

G

gambling, 46, 58, 134, 136, 145, 149, 150, 151

games, 65, 76, 77, 81, 134, 135, 141, 150

geriatrician, 25

glasses (reading), 4, 27, 105

grandchildren, 89, 90, 135, 161

gratitude, 56, 64, 116, 119

Greger, Dr. Michael, 19

grief (*also see* loss), 43, 60, 67

group exercise, 36

gym, 36-37, 149

gynecologist, 39, 102, 108, 109, 110

H

hair, 2-3, 42, 43, 47, 78, 102, 104, 105, 106, 112, 150

happiness, ix, 52, 59, 92, 140, 143, 155, 157, 188

Hay, Louise, xii, 63, 121

healthy aging, viii, 188

healthy eating, 18

hearing, 4, 27-28, 52, 93

heart attack, 26, 46, 71

heart disease, 15, 18, 25, 26, 41

high blood pressure, 18, 26, 41, 71

high cholesterol, 26, 71

high-intensity incidental physical activity (HIIPA), 35

high-intensity interval training (HIIT), 35, 53

hiking poles, 36

hoarding, 46, 128

hobbies, 67, 133, 139-140

Made in the USA
Middletown, DE
05 May 2021